Lose Weight,
Have More Energy
& Be Happier
in 10 Days

Take charge of your health
with the Master Cleanse

By Peter Glickman

Lose Weight, Have More Energy & Be Happier in 10 Days

© 2004, 2005 by Peter Glickman, Inc.
Published 2004, Second Edition 2005
Seventh printing, January 2008

Published by Peter Glickman, Inc., P.O Box 4984, Clearwater, Florida 33758-4984.

Editing, design and layout by Maggy Graham, Words & Pictures Press, Clearwater, Florida, 33763.

Illustrations by Ann Khotina.

Publisher's Cataloging-in-Publication Data

    Glickman, Peter
        Lose weight, have more energy & be happier in 10 days
     /Peter Glickman.—2nd ed.—Clearwater, FL: Peter Glickman,
    2005.
        158 p. 21.6 cm.
        ISBN 978-0-9755722-2-1

        1. Diet Therapy Popular Works. 2. Juice Diet. I. Title.

    RM237.G55 2004   615.854'22

Printed in the United States of America.

THE INFORMATION GIVEN IN THIS BOOK IS SOLELY FOR EDUCATIONAL PURPOSES. IT IS NOT INTENDED AS MEDICAL ADVICE. ANYONE WHO FOLLOWS IT DOES SO VOLUNTARILY.

Testimonials

"In August, I was diagnosed with a brain tumor. Most days are filled with headaches, dizziness, nausea, and some visual/balance problems. I've never had regular bowel movements and have always had bloating, gas, and several problems because of that. Since starting the cleanse, all those symptoms have disappeared and I've lost twelve pounds. I'm completely thrilled!! I go back to the neurologist Monday and can't wait to tell him all this.

"I plan to eat much healthier (after breaking the fast appropriately). I have more energy and clarity and feel more like myself.

"I just wanted to give my 'testimony.' This has been a godsend." — Angi Hardin

*****

"Peter, thanks again for the inspiration and information. I've lost about twelve to fourteen pounds. My waist is down two and one-half to three inches. I have to get another belt because the ones I have are all on the last notch. I've walked forty-six miles since starting, ridden my bike fourteen miles, and have worked each day (some better than others). I have a great feeling of peace, even though I hit some pretty stressful events head on. I am also giving serious thought to other work/life things. I guess the clarity and focus come from not eating. It is also a time to look at priorities." — Tony Bruno

*****

"I'd like to share my recent experience with regards to quitting smoking and cleansing at the same time.

"I have quit smoking using the patch about five times in the last twelve years, the longest period smoke-free being for a year and a half. Actually, since my son was born twelve years ago, I have spent most of that time either struggling to quit smoking or remain smoke-free. Quitting cigarettes was so physically and psychologically painful for me that I lived on the patch off and on for most of those twelve years. There was absolutely no way I could do it alone. Then, in July of this year I had a body scan that revealed spots on my right lung. Six months earlier I had had a mammogram that revealed a lump in one of my breasts. The doctor was 'keeping an eye on it.' Since I am forty-seven with a twelve-year-old son and I want to be around to watch him grow, I checked myself into a raw food cleansing/detox institute in the San Diego area. The experience was AMAZING.

"I asked them, 'Is it ok to wear the patch while going through the cleanse?' Their response to me was that I was trying to rid my body of toxins. Why would I want to put toxins in as I was trying to get them out? So I decided to leave the patches home and tough it out.

"We ate raw foods the first day and then juice-fasted for three days and then back to raw foods. I did this for three weeks. In the past when I quit smoking I would cough up tons of mucus and drain from my nose and eyes. My face would break out as my body tried to cleanse itself of all the toxins of cigarettes and all I wanted to do was eat. Of course there were also the TERRIBLE moods swings, irritability and anxiety. I was always sooooo miserable. But this time, quitting WHILE I cleansed made stopping smoking so different.

"At this institute they are big on cleansing the colon daily during the body cleanse, same as the Master Cleanse seems to be. I had absolutely NO coughing up of stuff, NO breakouts and, except for headache and fatigue the first couple of days, I felt better and more energetic than I have in years! I even started walking four miles a day and did this in about an hour and fifteen minutes. I COULDN'T BELIEVE IT!! I attribute this to the cleanse and the toxins being swiftly removed from my body through the colon, which alleviated all the negative side effects of stopping smoking. I say DEFINITELY try it without the patch while on the cleanse!!! My past experience says that I would STILL be on the patch right now while continuing to stay smoke-free.

"I am about to do the ten-day Master Cleanse (my first time) because through the holidays I've backslid on the raw and healthy food and am already feeling the difference and don't like it at all. I've experienced the 'good life' now and I don't want to lose it. By the way, a follow up mammogram after the cleanse revealed that my breast lump was gone. I attribute that to the cleanse also.

"Good luck to you. I hope this helps." —Betty Bridgeford

Table of Contents

A Huge Debt

The original book on the Master Cleanse is *The Master Cleanser* by Stanley Burroughs. Without Burroughs' work and that book, mankind would be significantly poorer. I owe a lot to Mr. Burroughs and if you do the Master Cleanse, you will also. His book describes the Master Cleanse along with Mr. Burroughs' views on disease and healing, some natural remedies, and some recipes for healthy food. It can be purchased from the Web Store of my website, www. TheMasterCleanse.com or by phone 727-524-6962. (It is published by Burroughs Books, 3702 S. Virginia St., Ste # G, Box # 346, Reno, NV 89502-6030.)

I am also in debt to all the wonderful people who participated on our bulletin board. Their encouragement, willingness to share, and insights have been and are wonderful, as you will see.

‖• NOTE: Throughout this book, an exclamation point to the left indicates the section is important.

Confession

I'm just an average Joe. I came upon the Master Cleanse because I was pig-headed enough to keep looking for a natural way to handle my failing health that would not cost me an arm and a leg and would not cause unwanted side effects. I just decided to keep looking until I found that way. Fortunately for me, I succeeded.

I am not a licensed health professional. I cannot diagnose and prescribe for anyone. However, I have seen that there are natural remedies that can help people regain and maintain their health. I have seen this information benefit more than a hundred people in one month alone. That is why I have written this book.

From reading some of the great healers of the past, I believe people can extend their lives and avoid illness and disease if they eat real, live food (raw fruits and vegetables, seeds and nuts), drink unpolluted and unfluoridated water, and clean their colons frequently.

I firmly believe that each person is responsible for his or her own health. A person who wants to be healthy, have energy and feel good must learn what is involved and apply it. You have to monitor what goes into your mouth, what exercise you do, what fresh air you breathe and, most important of all, what thoughts you think.

The good news is that valuable knowledge is available if you take the time to look for it and are willing to determine if it is true for you and your body. The reason you have to determine it for yourself is that each person's body is potentially different. For example, most people find penicillin valuable for killing bacteria. Some people are allergic and can die from it.

You are the only person who can make the determination of what is useful or not for you. Health professionals can give you valuable information and do other wonderful things, but ultimately, the buck stops with you. So you have to learn to use good judgment along with your experience, and that includes determining if the information in this book is useful to you.

Each person should seek the counsel of their health professional, and then use his or her own judgment. This caution applies to the information in this book and that posted on the website— www.TheMasterCleanse.com. In fact, this caution applies to any information in life.

If you are in ill health, have any disease or are taking any medications and want to do the Master Cleanse, consult your licensed healthcare professional first. Most especially, do not discontinue any medications without guidance from a licensed healthcare professional.

I think the Master Cleanse is great. You have to decide for yourself. I am only telling my story and some of the stories of the 110 people who did the Master Cleanse in January 2004 and posted their stories on the www.TheMasterCleanse.com bulletin board. If you have made the decision to do the Master Cleanse, congratulations for doing something really wonderful for yourself and your body!

Yours in health,
Peter Glickman

Introduction to the Second Edition

5 February 2005

In the seven months since the first edition, I have coached several hundred more people on the website bulletin board (www.TheMasterCleanse.com), learned a little more and want to share it with you.

For those curious to know what I've changed from the first edition, here they are:

1. I now recommend only using cayenne powder, not capsules.

2. According to a recent informal survey of 141 people who have done or are currently doing the Master Cleanse, hunger is experienced by about one out of four people while on the cleanse, rather than one out of twenty.

3. The same survey showed only one person out of 137 (that is how many answered this particular question) had any problem with their medication. And that lady only experienced the problem once out of the ten different times she has done the Master Cleanse!

4. I have had several questions about continuing birth control pills while on the Master Cleanse. I have now heard from several women that they have not had any problems and no one has mentioned any problem. So, I have included that information in this edition.

5. I corrected my instructions on breaking the fast. I said non-vegetarians could have vegetable soup for lunch the second day and Burroughs actually says not until dinner (supper) the second day.

6. I have added additional material in this Introduction on the widespread and growing problem of being overweight (pun intended), eating processed food, having a lack of energy, and being irritable and under stress; the reasons for this; and how the Master Cleanse and a raw fruit, vegetable, seed and nut diet can help in just days.

Being overweight has become far too common in America. According to a *Business Week* article, "Those Heavy Americans" (Gene Koretz, November 10, 2003), two-thirds of Americans are overweight. The market for weight loss products (low carbohydrate foods, diet programs, reducing supplements, etc.) is projected to surpass $150 billion by 2007. ("Weight Loss Market: Products, Services, Foods and Beverages," Business Communications Co., Inc., August 7, 2003)

Still worse, obesity or being overweight is projected to pass tobacco as the leading cause of preventable death in the United States this year (2005). ("Overweight and obesity: a major public health issue," U.S. Department of Health and Human Services, *Prevention Report* 2001) Those people it does not kill, it punishes, especially dating singles who want to be attractive to the opposite sex.

A look at our current culture might provide an explanation. SUPER SIZE ME is a very entertaining, feature-length color documentary film that shows what happens when the central character actually goes on a 30-day McDonald's-only diet. For 30 days, he eats breakfast, lunch and dinner at McDonald's. Nothing passes his lips that cannot be purchased at McDonald's. And whenever they ask him if he wants it super-sized, he must answer yes and eat it all.

At the beginning of the movie, we see him getting the results of various examinations by health care professionals. His results are all normal and he is given a clean bill of health. After three weeks, one doctor is shocked at how much worse his liver is and encourages him to go off the diet. Our "dieter" refuses. So, the doctor hands him a number for the hospital emergency room and insists he call if he experiences any symptoms of a heart attack! The doctor is shown in the film saying something along the lines of, "I would never have imagined that your diet could reduce your health this fast."

Not only does he gain more weight than expected, but we watch the deterioration in his complexion and mental attitude as well as learn about it from the results of his later blood tests. There are segments where he talks about his worsened mental attitude. His girlfriend, a vegan chef, also talks about his diminished sexual capability. (So, don't show the entire movie to your six year old without seeing it first. His girlfriend's description is not graphic, but you may have to answer questions you would rather not, if you show that part to your six year old.)

Another scene shows how children with learning and attitude problems change for the better when they are not fed processed food in their school cafeteria.

Toward the end of the movie, McDonald's French fries, a hamburger and a sandwich are put in separate glass domes along with a fresh-ground hamburger and hand-cut French fries from a local restaurant. The fresh-ground hamburger and hand-cut French fries decomposed as you would expect because they are not refrigerated. However, even without refrigeration, the McDonald's fries have no visible decomposition even after six weeks!

If they do not decompose like "nutritional" food, what does your body do with them? Your body uses the food you eat to nourish your body & blood, and build new cells. When you eat something that contains artificial preservatives, colors or flavors, your body has to neutralize it before it is eliminated. This is one of the jobs of the liver. When the liver receives too much to process at the time, it stores those toxins in fat cells in the liver to process later. When the liver runs out of room to store these, it releases them into the body and the body creates fat cells and stores the toxins in the body's fat cells until the toxins can be processed.

What keeps your liver strong and healthy? Blood from the colon is fed directly to the liver to nourish it. However, the body accumulates uneliminated toxins especially in the large intestine (colon), where blood has to filter through these toxins and poisons to get to the liver. At this point, the whole body is being fed "dirty blood." This is like trying to wash your hands in paint to get them clean. This is also what medicine refers to as "autointoxication": not "intoxication" as in happily relaxed, but as in self-poisoned. (*Tissue Cleansing Through Bowel Management*, by Dr. Bernard Jensen, DC, ND, Ph.D., 1980)

Symptoms of autointoxication include headaches, nausea, mental depression, irritability, stress, tension, tiredness, sluggishness, mental fogginess, indecision, insomnia, and susceptibility to other illnesses.

It is the toxins that Americans are eating and drinking that is causing the epidemic of overweight. Our bodies cannot handle the volume of toxins we consume on a daily basis.

Think processed food does not have toxins? In the article "Why McDonald's Fries Taste So Good" (*The Atlantic Monthly*, January 2001), the author, Eric Schlosser, says "About 90 percent of the money that Americans now spend on food goes to buy processed food." He goes on to say that the flavor is replaced with chemicals to add flavor. For example, there are approximately 350 different chemicals in high-quality artificial strawberry flavor.

Further in his article, he says, "One of the most widely used color additives ..., cochineal [pronounced koash-a-neil] extract ... is made from the [dried] bodies of [a small] female ... insect harvested mainly in Peru and the Canary Islands. The bug feeds on red cactus berries, and color from the berries accumulates in the females and their unhatched [young]. The insects are collected, dried, and ground into a pigment. It takes about 70,000 of them to produce a pound of carmine, which is used to make processed foods look pink, red, or purple. Dannon strawberry yogurt gets its color from carmine, and so do many frozen fruit bars, candies, and fruit fillings, and Ocean Spray pink-grapefruit juice drink." (His entire article is on the Internet at www.rense.com/general7/whyy.htm.)

The artificial sweetener Aspartame, also sold as NutraSweet, Equal, Equal Measure, and Spoonful, is another good example. The Food and Drug Administration has a system that permits people to report bad health reactions to food and drugs. According to David Rietz's website (www.dorway.com), in February of 1994, Aspartame accounted for more than 75% of **all** bad reactions reported!

A *Plane and Pilot* magazine article (January 1990) on food additives explained that diet soft drinks are sweetened artificially by Aspartame (NutraSweet and Equal). Aspartame contains 10% methanol, a poison, that is released at temperatures above 86° or if left on the shelf for a long time.

The article goes on to say that methanol destroys the brain a little at a time. Immediate effects can either be severe (epileptic seizures, blindness, or chest palpitations) or less noticeable (blurred vision, bright flashes, tunnel vision, ringing or buzzing in ears, migraine headaches, dizziness, loss of equilibrium, or lip and mouth reactions). It reports on an Air Force pilot who directly traced the patterns of tremors and seizures he suffered for two years to his consuming NutraSweet in beverages. His medical problems ceased when he quit drinking NutraSweet.

By the way, on 27 June 1996, without public notice, the FDA removed all restrictions from Aspartame, allowing it to be used in everything, including all heated and baked goods. (webhome.idirect.com/ ~wolfnowl/aspartame.htm)

Even when you go on a diet and eat less, forcing the body to burn fat, as soon as you go off the diet, the fat returns. The body must create more fat cells to protect itself from the toxins. The only effective way to eliminate the fat is to eliminate the toxins. This is why the Master Cleanse is so effective for not only losing weight, but also increasing energy and making people happier. In the recent informal survey of 141 people who have done or are on the Master Cleanse, about 80% of them report having more energy and more than 90% report being happier! This should be no surprise since toxins give you headaches, make you fell tired and irritable, and cause aches and pains. And the Master Cleanse, according to its developer, Stanley Burroughs, not only cleanses the colon, but also the liver, kidneys and other organs and glands.

A raw vegetable, fruit, seed and nut diet will also detoxify you, although more slowly. But in my experience, very, very few people can simply switch to eating 100% raw. However, a great many people can do the Master Cleanse and, having eliminated some cravings, eat a greater percentage of raw food than before. This is supported by the above survey, which showed that people on average rated their diet after the Master Cleanse as being somewhat healthier than before the Master Cleanse.

How did I learn about the Master Cleanse and the raw food diet? Well, in the fall of 1998, I was a successful executive of a small local software company. I was coming home at 6:30 pm and dropping into bed, so tired I did not even eat dinner. I would not get up until it was 8 a.m. and time to go to work again. No one at work, except my wife, knew I was not doing well. At home, however, my excessive tiredness and short temper were inescapable. Worse, food had become my enemy. No matter what I ate, I felt sick afterward.

About a year and a half before, I had been tested and discovered I had enough mercury in my body to interfere with normal system function. Apparently, it was finally getting to me. I sought a local doctor to do a mercury detoxification program on me and before he put me on that program, he gave me a thorough checkup.

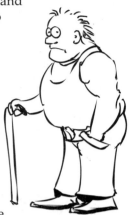

The blood test came back with alarming numbers. My fasting blood sugar was in the range of diabetics (157), the fats that circulate in the bloodstream and are stored in the fat tissue (triglycerides) were really, really high (1160) and my cholesterol was in the same scary place (482). The doctor scared me badly enough that I radically changed my diet. I eliminated any sweet food including sweet fruits, sweet vegetables, etc. and added the vitamins and minerals that Adele Davis recommended for diabetics in her book, *Let's Get Well*. This was in addition to the mercury detoxification program, which included super greens (a combination of spirulina, blue green algae, alfalfa, wheatgrass and other greens).

Fortunately, in the next four months, my tests all returned to normal levels and I could go back to eating the standard American diet of too many fats, too much sugar, very few raw vegetables or fruits, and lots of processed food. Three years later in May 2002, I had another checkup and this time, although my fasting blood sugar was fine (108), my blood fats were the second highest the doctor had ever seen (1921) and my cholesterol was so scary (525) that he had his office call me in immediately to be put on a prescription. I listened to him, filled it immediately and tried it for three days. It gave me a headache and bad dreams. I figured I had licked the blood sugar problem with nutrition, why couldn't I lick the cholesterol problem the same way?

By May 2002, my wife had been eating a 100% raw fruit, vegetable, nuts and seeds diet for more than six months. She was looking healthy and radiant, had lost weight, had plenty of energy and felt great. I tried to ignore how healthy she was for several months, but after the prescription fiasco, I decided I would go on the same diet and see what happened. I wasn't feeling as bad as I had before the mercury detoxification; I still didn't realize my road rage was connected to my health; and I still didn't have the energy I used to have. But wasn't that normal?

When I started the raw vegetarian diet in May 2002, I weighed over 230 pounds. I wore pants with a size 40 waist, which were tight. Over the next six months, I lost more than thirty pounds and was now fitting into size 37 pants. But more importantly I felt great and had lots of energy. Road rage became a thing of the past. People who saw me asked what I was doing to look so much better.

In December 2002, I began wondering if I should do some kind of cleanse. I had done a liver/gall bladder cleanse some years before and wondered if perhaps another type of cleanse or a whole series of different cleanses was something I needed at this point. So when I discovered the Master Cleanse by Stanley Burroughs at the end of December, I decided to do it starting in January 2003.

The Master Cleanse changed my life. I did it for 20 days and lost 23 pounds. Much, much more important, I felt fabulous and was now able to work 10 – 14 hour days with no strain at all and I was happier than I'd been in years and years!

My wife also did the Master Cleanse. So did my twenty-seven year old son and his girl friend, as well as a friend I hadn't talked to for three years. When he heard I'd lost over fifty pounds and felt great, he said he wanted to do it and didn't care what it was. He discovered that on the Master Cleanse, he could still walk his six miles a day and he had enough energy to also ride his bike another four miles most days as well.

I already had a website for raw food and decided to add information on the Master Cleanse and a bulletin board so people who had questions could have a place to get answers from those who had done the Master Cleanse. From there, it was only a small step to see if we could get 100 people to do the Master Cleanse in January 2004 to start the year. Amazingly, with only one story in a local monthly health magazine and word of mouth, we ended up with more than 110 people doing it! Last month, January 2005, we had 218 people doing the cleanse in January!

Did you keep the weight off? That's a question I'm frequently asked. Well, I finished my first Master Cleanse on 24 January 2003 weighing 175 pounds. As I write this, February 2005, I weigh the same. More importantly, I am in vibrant good health and it shows.

I wish you the best,
Peter Glickman

Part II:

How to Do the Master Cleanse

Shopping List*:

The Master Cleanser book
- About 40 large lemons or 80 limes or a combination (organic preferred). Only enough for five days (half the amount) at a time or they spoil.
- At least 80 fl. oz. Organic Grade B Maple Syrup (usually sold in 32 fl. oz. bottles = 2.5 bottles)
- 1/2 pound non-iodized Sea Salt (I recommend Light Grey Celtic Sea Salt)
- 2.5 ounces of cayenne pepper (powdered hot red pepper)
- A box of herbal laxative tea bags
- At least five gallons (640 fl. oz.) spring or purified water (not fluoridated†) for the lemonade and another 3 gallons and a pint (400 fl. oz.) for the salt water flush and a cup of laxative tea

* These quantities are based on a 10-day cleanse with 8 glasses of lemonade a day, which is what I averaged. Stanley Burroughs says to drink 6 – 12 glasses a day. So, you may need to adjust the quantities.

† Fluorine is about as poisonous as lead or arsenic and was used for decades as rat poison. It is very injurious to human health and several studies have shown it to increase the risk of cancer.

The Nitty Gritty

1.   The Master Cleanse should be done for at least ten days. Burroughs says it can be done for forty or more days. I've personally done it more than nine times from ten to twenty-eight days (and once for

three days) —all within the last two years. Burroughs is right about ten days being the minimum. The three-day Master Cleanse left me feeling as though nothing had been accomplished. I can hear you saying, "Ten days?! Is he crazy?" Amazingly, you will not be hungry and you will have more energy than you felt before the Master Cleanse. (By actual count, six out of one hundred twenty people told me they were genuinely hungry.)

In addition to my own longer Master Cleanses, I know of three other people who have done it for twenty days. All of us found that there were spiritual gains after eight or ten days: a clarity of purpose, a sense of focus, a feeling of well being, and a discovery that our natural emotion is one of cheerful satisfaction.

Burroughs says the best sign that the Master Cleanse is complete is a clear, pink tongue. Your tongue will definitely get coated and turn white and possibly other colors. (For pictures of various tongue coatings, visit the links in the topic "Tongue Coating" below.) Not everyone continues until their tongue is clear and pink. Most stop at ten days regardless of tongue color. However, ten days is long enough to make a major change in your weight, health and mental outlook.

2.   Before you go to bed, drink one cup of herbal laxative tea the evening before you start the Master Cleanse. You can buy this in most health food stores. There are two types I am aware of: pure senna tea and combinations of senna with other herbs. Senna is a strong herb that promotes intestinal contractions that cause elimination. Some people find senna causes uncomfortably strong contractions. Others have no problem with pure senna. You can also make half a cup of pure senna and then add half a cup of warm or hot water to make it a full cup.

I personally did not have any problem with senna until my third Master Cleanse. Then I felt uncomfortably strong contractions and switched to a combination tea. Occasionally, when I run out of the combination, I'll make half a cup and dilute it. Two of the combination teas are Smooth Move and Get Regular.

I have been asked (rarely) if senna is addictive or will cause damage. I have never seen or heard of damage or addiction with any of the people who have done the Master Cleanse that I am aware of (more than 100). Perhaps 10% have reported uncomfortable cramps. In my experience, the cramps have disappeared when the salt water or lemonade is drunk and can be avoided by using the combination teas. The senna box warns not to give it to children or to drink more than two cups per day. The combination box says not to drink more than four cups per day and half that for children from six to twelve years old.

3.   Upon awakening on the first morning and each morning thereafter on the Master Cleanse, drink a quart of water with two level teaspoons of NON-IODIZED SEA SALT. Drink it all at once or as close to that as you can. Use NON-IODIZED SEA SALT because it will be easier to drink than bleached pure white table salt. The other reason to use NON-IODIZED SEA SALT is that it contains vital trace minerals that your body needs. Do not drink any lemonade for a half hour after drinking the salt water. I personally recommend Light Grey Celtic Sea Salt, which can be found at most health food stores.

Approximately one half to one hour after drinking the salt water, you will have several urges to eliminate. Stay near the toilet. These eliminations will generally continue for one half to one hour after they start. You will need to plan your day accordingly.

Some people have trouble with drinking the salt water. Be sure you stir the salt water so the salt is evenly distributed in the drink just before you drink it. It will be easier to drink and it is more effective. I believe it is very important to include it. So try everything you can. My wife found it helpful to drink it through a straw or to count the number of swallows as you drink it. Do not add anything to the salt water to make it taste better. Stay with the program. If you find that you absolutely cannot drink the salt water, Burroughs says you can drink another cup of herbal laxative tea in the morning instead. However, the laxative stimulates the muscles of the intestinal wall to contract and mechanically move the waste through. The salt water flushes whatever loose waste is in the digestive tract and the salt also helps to dissolve the mucus and waste.

Many people have noticed that it is much easier to drink the salt water flush on later days of a cleanse. I believe this may be because the body reacts more dramatically when it has more mucus in the system and, as that gets cleaned out, the body has less reaction to the salt water flush.

The reason for two teaspoons of salt is to increase the weight (specific gravity) of the salt water until it matches the weight of blood. Specific gravity is how heavy the substance is compared to an equal volume of water. When the salt water and the blood are the same, the body

21

will treat the salt water as though it were blood, not absorb it from the digestive system, and will just "flush" the salt water through the system instead of absorbing it. You might occasionally need to increase the amount of salt in the water to make the flush effective.

People who have recently been on the Atkins diet or any heavy meat and dairy diet may need two or three days before the flush produces eliminations. This is because meat and dairy are frequently hard to digest and build up waste that clogs the colon.

4. Mix and drink six to twelve glasses of lemonade each day of the Master Cleanse. Here's the recipe:

2 tbsp. (1 fl. oz.) of fresh squeezed lemon or lime juice,

2 tbsp. (1 fl. oz.) of grade B organic maple syrup,

1/10th tsp. of cayenne (hot red) pepper, and

8 fl. oz. of spring or purified water or substitute 10 fl. oz. of fresh sugar cane juice for the water and maple syrup. Do not use fluoridated water.

The enzymes in the lemon break down the layers of old waste in the colon. Although the lemon is acidic, it becomes alkaline when digested and the alkalinity helps neutralize the acidity of the toxic wastes. Try to get organic lemons from your local health food store, if possible, as they contain more minerals than non-organic ones. The lemon juice must be fresh squeezed, not bottled. The enzymes begin to break down within hours and heating kills them completely. If you must prepare the drinks for most of the day—for taking to work, for example—prepare only that much and make fresh lemonade when you get home for the rest of the day. To make up more than one day's lemonade at one time or to try to save the squeezed lemon juice for another day will lose a great deal of the potency of the lemons.

The maple syrup supplies the sugar for energy and more importantly, it supplies the needed minerals. The darker the syrup, the more minerals. A is lighter than B. So try to get B if possible, but any organic grade will do. The reason for organic is that some companies use formaldehyde in the process of tapping the trees. Organic grade B maple syrup can be found in most health food stores.

Cayenne pepper has many wonderful properties. In the Master Cleanse, it is used to break up the mucus and dilate the blood vessels, thus accelerating the detoxification process. If you can increase the amount of cayenne in your drinks, you will accelerate your Master Cleanse.

● Do not take cayenne in capsules. Dr. Richard Schulze, a Master Herbalist, reports that people who take cayenne capsules do not receive much of the benefit of the cayenne. The nerve endings in the mouth respond almost instantly to send blood throughout the body. This whole process is missed if you take capsules.

In addition, gelatin is made from boiled skin, bones and tendons. That is a lot of digestive work — especially when you are not eating food to give your digestive system a chance to cleanse itself. So, taking cayenne capsules should not be done.

If you "can't drink cayenne" it is usually because you took too much at some time before this. Start with just a sprinkle and gradually increase it as you tolerate more. Decide to learn to take cayenne. It is wonderful for your health.

5.   In addition to the above, you may drink as much spring or purified water as you wish and occasionally some mint tea for a change. Do not use fluoridated water.

6.   Nothing else is eaten or drunk on the Master Cleanse.

● 7. Breaking the Master Cleanse diet correctly is **very important!** I have heard one second-hand story of someone going straight to overeating ribs and dessert who had serious medical problems. I do not know if this story is true, but I know personally that diving immediately back into a bad diet will make you feel very sick for a few hours.

If you usually eat meat, cooked food, dairy, etc., to break the fast Burroughs says to drink fresh squeezed orange juice for the first and second day with homemade vegetable soup for dinner the second evening eating mostly broth and a few vegetables — no bread or crackers. The third day should be orange juice in the morning, more of the homemade vegetable soup for lunch and salads, fruits and/or vegetables for dinner. Begin eating your usual food the fourth day, although Burroughs recommends lemonade or fruit juice for breakfast on a continuing basis and a vegetarian diet as the best means of preserving life-long health.

If you are a raw vegetarian, he tells you to drink fresh orange juice the first, second and morning of the third day. For lunch on the third day have raw fruit, with a raw fruit or vegetable salad for dinner. After that, eat normally. I used to find the orange juice too rich for me and chose to drink grapefruit juice instead when coming off the Master Cleanse.

If you have gas or digestive upset when breaking the fast, Burroughs says to continue the Master Cleanse a few more days.

● Detox Symptoms—the Good, the Bad and the Ugly

Detox symptoms are what you feel when toxins are mobilized, but not yet eliminated. They are a double-edged sword. Detox symptoms are a milestone in the detoxifying process. They indicate you are mobilizing and eliminating toxins. Unfortunately, they do not make you feel good.

It is important for someone on the Master Cleanse to know what detox symptoms are and that they typically go away after the next morning's eliminations. It is next to impossible to go through ten consecutive days of cravings or tiredness with no relief in sight, but when you know those feelings will be gone with tomorrow's eliminations, anyone can make it through the Master Cleanse.

I divide detox symptoms into these classes:

1. **Cravings**. When your body is detoxifying from incompletely digested ribs, hamburgers, pizza, cheese, etc., you will crave whatever is being detoxified. Paavo Airola discusses this concept on page 153 in his book *How to Get Well*.

2. **Irritability, boredom, etc.** The irritability of dieters is common knowledge. Among the reasons for this is that reduced eating allows the body to detox and one of the symptoms of detoxification is irritability. In this class of symptoms, I also include boredom, anxiety, wanting to "just chew something," and wanting to quit the Master Cleanse. It is quite remarkable how the next day's eliminations can change your attitude toward the Master Cleanse. When you get to Day 8 or so, you may discover for yourself that your natural mood is positive and cheerful. I have a friend in Georgia who told me how surprised he was that he was able to

stay so upbeat during the Master Cleanse in the face of some serious problems.

3. **Headaches and other aches.** Very few people on the Master Cleanse get headaches or other aches: in my experience perhaps 5% or less. Those who get headaches have heavy caffeine habits before going cold turkey on the Master Cleanse. These headaches lasted three to five days. Other people may have aches and pains from previous illnesses for a few days before these aches and pains disappear a few days later. A friend had very severe hemorrhoids previous to the Master Cleanse. They appeared a few days after he started and went away a few days later. It was his impression that they would not be back.

4. **Tiredness.** It should not be strange that the toxins which age you and drain your energy should make you tired. They do until they are eliminated. That is why both the Agitator and the Rinse Cycle (See below.) are so important.

5. **Burning bowel movements.** Toxins and other waste are acidic. I have found that when I eliminate old waste and other toxins, my bowel movements are actually hot. During my first Master Cleanse, my eliminations actually burned. I have also noticed that when I have serious detox symptoms as listed above, my eliminations the next morning are typically hot.

Occasionally, someone will ask if it is the cayenne that burns. While cayenne in large quantities can temporarily cause hot bowel movements, this does not explain how — on a constant dose of cayenne — one can suddenly experience hot bowel movements after several days of normal temperatures. No, I am convinced it is the acidic toxins being eliminated.

● "How About Only Five Days? Can We Make a Deal?"

Burroughs says to do the Master Cleanse for at least ten days at a time. Many people have asked if they could do it for less. My experience has shown that the days with the greatest chances for detox symptoms—remember, they are the milestones of progress—are the second, third, sixth or seventh and fourteenth or fifteenth (for those that go that long). The second and third days are fairly obvious. That's when the recent waste is being eliminated and thus is causing detox symptoms —cravings, irritability, etc. Notice that the sixth/seventh and fourteenth/fifteenth are approximately seven days apart. At a talk given by Victoria Boutenko, a raw vegetarian speaker and writer, she showed a video of a live blood analysis that showed the clumping of red blood cells when people ate cooked food. She said it took seven days for the red blood cells to un-clump. Perhaps there is a seven-day cycle in the body that is triggered by the Master Cleanse. At any rate, I've noticed that the biggest benefits in mental clarity, serenity and focus come for most people after Day 8. The moral of the story? Stick with it for at least ten days, just like Burroughs says.

● The Agitator and the Rinse Cycle

The Master Cleanse is designed to do two things: first to detoxify the body (remove toxins/poisons from the cells and organs in which they are embedded)—The Agitator—and then to eliminate those toxins from the body before they can be reabsorbed and poison the body once again—the Rinse Cycle. Just as a washing machine must incorporate both of those to be effective, so must any good cleanse.

Not eating any solid food permits your body to direct all of its digestive energy toward removing toxins from the cells and organs in which they are embedded. This process is aided by the six to twelve ten-ounce glasses of "lemonade" per day that you will drink on the Master Cleanse. The lemon juice helps to neutralize the acidic wastes and loosen them from where they are stored, and the cayenne pepper increases the blood flow to areas to be detoxified by dilating the blood vessels. The final part of the Agitator is the herbal laxative tea which stimulates the muscular contractions in the intestines, which "agitates" the contents and moves them toward final elimination.

Once the old toxic waste has been mobilized, you need the Rinse Cycle to eliminate it before it is reabsorbed. After the stomach has reduced the food you have eaten to a semi-liquid form, your body pushes it through the intestines where it absorbs what you have given it for nourishment. If the walls of the intestines are coated with years of waste, all daily nutrients must be absorbed through this coating and some of the old putrefied waste is carried into the blood stream.

Sadly, most "civilized" people tend to overeat, and to choose those things which are the most difficult to digest, such as meat and cheese. The "end" result of this kind of diet over decades is an accumulation of toxic waste, which is then re-absorbed into the blood. (You can read more about this in the excellent books by Dr. Norman W. Walker, such as *Colon Health: The Key to a Vibrant Life*, or *Become Younger*. Dr. Walker, by the way, lived well past 100 years of age, was mentally sharp and physically fit throughout his life, and is credited with the statement, "Death begins in the colon.")

The salt water flush is the Rinse Cycle and therefore vital. Burroughs does say that if you cannot drink the salt water flush in the morning, you should drink the laxative tea both evening and morning. (Take care not to drink more than two cups per day of pure senna tea or four cups per day of tea with 50% senna.) However, I believe that the agitator action of the laxative tea is different than the flushing action of the salt water flush and encourage people to do the salt water flush if at all possible. You would not wash your clothes in a washing machine with only an agitator and no rinse cycle, so why clean your digestive tract without a rinse cycle?

● Some People Need to Take It Easy

If you mobilize more toxins than you can daily eliminate, you will feel bad. People with lots of toxins need to take it easy at first. This gives rise to two questions:

1. Who needs to take it easy?

2. What does "take it easy" actually mean?

Here are indicators that you might need to take it easy:

1. **Seriously overweight**—The body stores toxins in fat cells when it runs out of room in the liver. Serious overweight indicates there may be lots of toxins and waste to eliminate.

2. **Multiple-year history of medical drugs**—Antibiotics every few years for infections are probably not much to worry about. Sleeping pills every night for ten years is another situation. If you are on or have had heavy psychiatric drugs, chemotherapy, etc. you should definitely check with your health professional.

3. **Allergic to many things** — Alternative medicine equates allergies with toxic reactions. If you are only allergic to bananas, that is probably not too serious. If you are allergic to fifteen things, you need to take it easy.

● Taking It Easy

For those people who have decided they should take it easy, I recommend the following:

1. Drink only the minimum six drinks of lemonade each day.

2. Be sure to drink the herbal laxative tea every evening.

3. Drink enough additional water so that you have drunk at least one ounce of water or lemonade for each two pounds of body weight each day.

4. Be sure to do the salt water flush as given each morning.

5. Take long, soaking hot baths to draw out toxins (not in fluoridated water).

6. Immediately discontinue the Master Cleanse if any detox symptoms do not disappear or lessen with the next day's eliminations.

7. If you did have to discontinue the Master Cleanse, do a slower cleanse by eating fresh raw vegetables, fruits, nuts and seeds for a month or so. (Even then, you may have to eat some bread or cooked rice to slow down the detox.)

The reasoning behind the recommendations above is to detoxify very lightly, but use the maximum amount of elimination methods so that whatever toxins are mobilized are quickly eliminated before being reabsorbed. Remember, you can do the Master Cleanse several times. So, do not push it.

If you have any doubts, discuss your concerns with a health professional.

Headaches

As I pointed out in **Detox Symptoms—The Good, the Bad and the Ugly**, people who have heavy daily caffeine habits — coffee, tea, soda with caffeine, etc.— typically have bad headaches when they go cold turkey on the Master Cleanse. Realize it is the caffeine habit you are kicking and persevere. It does not make any sense to me to go off the Master Cleanse with its enhanced elimination in order to attempt to kick the habit without the enhanced elimination procedures. The longest I have known someone to have a headache was four days. Keep in mind if you have a headache for more than a day or so and never had a caffeine habit, this may signal other problems that you should not ignore. Therefore, you should quickly discover the cause.

Hunger

I originally thought that hunger during the Master Cleanse was very rare as only a few people on the first January cleanse (2004) mentioned it. However, in a recent survey I did of 141 people who have done or are doing the Master Cleanse, about one quarter mentioned being hungry at some time during the cleanse. Fortunately for most people, drinking more lemonade or water (8 – 10 oz.) eliminates the hunger in about ten minutes.

It is also possible these people confused hunger with cravings. The way to distinguish between hunger and cravings is to ask yourself if you are interested in eating an apple, some carrots or a fresh green salad. If you are interested in those, you are hungry. If they do not interest you, but you are interested in ribs, French fries, a hamburger, etc., you are experiencing cravings. As cravings are a detox symptom, they will diminish or go away entirely after your next morning's eliminations if you are doing the Master Cleanse as written.

❗ When It Is Not All Coming Out as Planned

Not having any bowel movements? Here is a checklist to help you. However, keep in mind that you may only have watery movements for several days. As long as something is coming out, watery or not, do not worry. The lemonade and not eating will dissolve the old waste and toxins.

1. Are you putting at least two level TEASPOONS of sea salt in the water each morning?

2. Are you mixing two tablespoons (one ounce) of FRESH-SQUEEZED—not bottled—lemon juice into each drink or using these proportions for each batch and only mixing one day at a time?

3. Are you adding cayenne pepper to taste with each drink?

4. Are you drinking one cup of laxative tea each morning AS WELL AS each evening and the salt water flush to encourage more elimination? (Note: Discontinue the extra cup in the morning after you get things going.)

5. Are you eating or drinking ANYTHING else but lemonade, water, salt water, laxative herb tea and occasional mint tea?

6. Before this cleanse, did you have only one or two BMs per week? Being constipated before the Master Cleanse might mean a little longer before you see results.

7. Are you on any constipating medications? I am NOT suggesting you quit taking any prescribed medications. But they may delay the results of the Master Cleanse.

❗ The 12 Most Common Pitfalls

More than eight hundred people are members of The Raw Food Site / Master Cleanse Bulletin Board (www.TheMasterCleanse.com) as I write this in January 2005. Many, many more people read this bulletin board and ask questions as guests without becoming members. As the day-to-day moderator, I have read the majority of their questions and answers and posted more than six hundred answers of my own in the last year alone! These 12 pitfalls are the most common. If you can avoid these, you will multiply your chances for success by 12 times.

1. Not getting all the correct written information before starting the cleanse

I know. You think I'm saying this just because I want to sell my book. Well, I do want to sell my book. But that's not why I'm saying this. Remember the children's game "telephone" where you whisper a message from one person to another? The person who told you how to do it may or may not have remembered all the important information. They may not have the same concerns that you have. So they don't mention something important to you.

There are so many strange alterations. I can't remember them all. But they have one thing in common. They won't get the great results that everyone else gets by following Stanley Burroughs' instructions. When you verbally tell your friend what you remember about the cleanse, you may be setting them up for a failure. And they may not remember exactly what you said either. I wish I had a dollar for everyone who says, "Oh… 2 **TEASPOONS** of sea salt in the salt water flush. I was trying to do it with 2 tablespoons!"

I've seen real people on the bulletin board talk about adding soy sauce to the salt water flush so it's like soup. (Soy sauce is protein and requires almost as much digestion as hamburger!) Another asked how many of the glasses of orange juice or vegetable soup are permitted each afternoon on the cleanse. Her friend described it, but didn't remember how many each day. Another woman talked about how she tried to handle her hunger with vegetable soup each afternoon!

To best help your friends, either give them the book or tell them to go buy it. They'll value it more. And they'll get the straight scoop. Their significant other might pick it up and help them or join them, too!

2. Not knowing what "detox" means

"Detox" is short for detoxify — meaning to eliminate toxins (poisons). It comes from "de-" meaning down or away, "toxin" meaning poison, and "-ify" meaning to make or do. So, "detoxify" means to make poisons come out or away (from the body). The toxins in our case are substances that your body can't absorb and use to rebuild the body.

They actually harm your body's cells making you fat, tired, irritable, sick or, in extreme cases, dead.

So, when a person detoxifies, or detoxes, she or he is mobilizing the toxins stored in various places and eliminating them. When they are mobilized, the person may become tired, feel pain or aches, be irritable, develop rashes, etc. These symptoms (signs showing that something else exists) tell you that toxins have been mobilized. Next, they need to be eliminated. Once they are eliminated, you will feel better than before. This is the whole purpose of a cleanse. To eliminate toxins so that you feel and are healthier than before you started the cleanse.

3. Not knowing the detox symptoms

I divide detox symptoms into five categories:

Cravings — You crave what your body is detoxifying. If you have some incompletely digested ribs, hamburgers, pizza, cheese, etc., you will crave it when your body mobilizes it until it's eliminated. This is very important to understand because cravings will be gone with tomorrow's eliminations. It's important to know you won't have to live with a constant yearning for pizza, bread, or Thai duck.

Irritability — The irritability of dieters is common knowledge. One of the reasons for this is that reduced eating allows the body to detox and one of the symptoms of detoxifying is irritability. In this class of symptoms, I also include boredom, anxiety, wanting to "just chew something," and wanting to quit the Master Cleanse. It is quite remarkable how the next day's eliminations can change your attitude toward the Master Cleanse. When you get to day eight or so, you will discover for yourself that your natural mood is positive and cheerful. Anything less is a detox symptom. I have a friend in Georgia who told me how surprised he was that he was able to stay so upbeat during the Master Cleanse in the face of some serious problems.

Headaches and other aches — Very few people on the Master Cleanse get headaches or other aches. In my experience it is only one person out of 20. Those who get headaches usually have heavy coffee or cola caffeine habits. These headaches usually last from two to four days. Other people may have aches and pains from previous illnesses that flare up for a few days before they disappear. A friend of mine had very severe hemorrhoids previous to the Master Cleanse. They appeared a few days after he started and went away a few days later. It was his impression that they would not be back.

Tiredness — It should be obvious that the toxins, which age you and drain your energy, would make you tired. They do.

Burning bowel movements — Toxins and other waste are acidic. I have found that when I eliminate old waste and other toxins, my bowel movements are actually hot. During my first Master Cleanse, my eliminations actually burned. I have also noticed that when I have serious detox symptoms as listed above, my eliminations the next morning are typically hot. Someone suggested that the cayenne pepper from the cleanse is what makes the eliminations hot. This doesn't make sense to me because I may go several days before I have a hot elimination and the cayenne was constant.

Detox symptoms are a double-edged sword — you want them and you don't. They indicate you're mobilizing and eliminating toxins, but you don't feel good while you have them.

4. Not knowing that detox symptoms will usually be gone or lessened with the next day's eliminations

The detox symptoms above usually go away or at least lessen with the next day's eliminations. This is vital to understand because very few people can make it through ten straight days of cravings. But if you know those feelings will only last one more day, you can make it through all ten days of the Master Cleanse easily.

Too often, I hear of people quitting because they were discouraged and thought nothing was happening. First, their discouragement was a detox symptom — a sign something **was** happening. Second, they were only one morning away from feeling great and knowing they could do it. So, you can see how important it is to know about this pitfall.

The reverse of this is also important. If you are feeling sick and it doesn't go away or lessen after a few days, it is probably not a detox symptom. What then? If it's serious, consult your licensed health care practitioner. If it's not, either come off the cleanse and handle it or handle it as you think best.

5. Not doing all the elimination actions every day

The pitfall above (not knowing that detox symptoms will usually be gone or lessen with the next day's eliminations) depends on doing all the elimination actions each day.

I think of The Master Cleanse as having two parts: the "Agitator" and the "Rinse Cycle." The agitator in a washing machine loosens the dirt. The rinse cycle then washes it away. These two actions combine to get clothes really clean.

When you cleanse, your digestive system begins to eliminate old waste. The lemon juice helps to dissolve it. The herbal laxative tea encourages the muscles in the intestines to contract in waves. These contractions loosen the old waste from the intestine walls and move it along and out. These are all "Agitator" actions.

The "rinse cycle" is composed of the salt water flush each morning and drinking at least one ounce of water or lemonade each day for every two pounds of body weight. For example, if you weigh 200 pounds, you should be drinking at least 100 ounces of water or lemonade per day. The 32-ounce salt water flush doesn't count as it just washes through the system and is not absorbed.

The "agitator" actions are loosening (mobilizing) the old waste with its toxins. If you don't drink enough lemonade and water and don't do the salt water flush each morning, the toxins are not going to be eliminated quickly. They will be reabsorbed. You will feel tired, sick, achy and may have cravings. All this can be prevented or minimized by ensuring you do all the elimination ("rinse cycle") actions each day without fail.

[Burroughs does say if you can't do the salt water flush first thing in the morning, you must drink the herbal laxative tea every morning as well. However, I believe that isn't as good as doing the salt water flush each morning. So, if you absolutely can't do the salt water flush, do the laxative tea in the morning as well. But if you can do the salt water flush, force yourself. (Yes, I know it's difficult. But it does get easier...honest.)

When people tell me they are tired or frustrated the first thing I check is whether they are doing all their elimination actions each day. If they are, all will be well tomorrow. If they aren't, they better start doing them before they feel worse.

6. Not knowing the worst days are usually 2, 3, & 7

I believe it is important to know which days are going to be the worst. For one thing, you will know that the entire Master Cleanse will not be that difficult. For another, you can look forward to better days. (By the way, people usually gain mental clarity starting with day 8.)

It's amazing how many people quit on 2, 3, and 7! (Occasionally someone will be off by a day and have day 1 be the worst or day 6.) In addition to not knowing which days are the worst, they usually don't know the detox symptoms and that they go away if the elimination actions are done each day.

I have observed that the body detoxes in seven-day cycles. When I did my 20-day cleanse, days 2, 3, 7, and 14 were the worst. I just recently finished a 28-day cleanse, but days 21 and 28 were fine. So, it's not *always* every 7 days, but very frequently it is the case. Of course I've done nine cleanses in the last two years and each one gets easier.

7. Confusing cravings with hunger

How do you tell the difference? If you really want a hamburger, but you'd turn down a green salad, it's a craving. Why does it make any difference? When you realize you are feeling cravings, not hunger, you know they are just detox symptoms. And you can make it to the next day.

8. Not drinking more lemonade or water when you feel hungry

Only one person in four reports any hunger on this cleanse. After checking to see if they are craving some food in particular, I tell them to drink more lemonade or water when they feel hungry. And their hunger usually disappears.

9. Eating or drinking anything else except lemonade, salt water, herbal laxative tea or mint tea while on the cleanse (except items prescribed by licensed health professionals)

A lady once posted to The Master Cleanse Bulletin Board that she kept feeling hungry. When I asked her to tell me exactly what she was doing, she told me she was drinking vegetable soup each afternoon! Of course, this was creating new cravings to torture her every day! So, rather than being done with cravings after the third day, she was continuing her cravings every single day of the cleanse!

Other people have asked about taking additional items, such as vitamins, supplements, chewing gum, sweetener for the tea, herbs, etc.

Hundreds of thousands of people have done The Master Cleanse since it was developed by Stanley Burroughs. It works. Just as written. The lemonade and maple syrup have all the necessary vitamins, minerals and calories to support the body for the duration of the cleanse.

10. Not using fresh-squeezed lemon juice

I'm not saying you have to freshly squeeze the lemon (or lime) juice for each glass one at a time. If you've got to go to work all day, you're going to have to make up enough for one day ahead of time. But try to make the last drink or two with freshly squeezed lemon juice after you get home.

What I am saying is do **not** use bottled, processed, or yesterday's juice. It's the enzymes (substances that encourage chemical changes) in the lemon juice that make it effective. These enzymes become less effective over time.

By using freshly squeezed juice, you will keep is as effective as possible to help dissolve the old waste.

11. Going to social events during the first 7 days

Something wonderful happens on day 8. People usually discover that they can cook for others or go out to eat with others and not go off the cleanse. (Usually, they gain mental clarity, too.)

However, before then, don't tempt yourself. Especially on days 2, 3 and 7.

12. Being so focused on losing pounds that you don't notice you're losing inches

My wife discovered something interesting. She kept track of her measurements each day as well as her weight. A couple times her weight didn't change. But she noticed that she was losing inches in places she wanted. Others talk about being able to fit into clothes they couldn't wear before even though they hadn't lost many pounds.

Part III

Your Master Cleanse Journal

Date Started: _____ Weight: _____

Measurements: Chest: _____ Waist: _____ Hips: _____ Thighs: _____

Energy level on a scale of one to ten (one being the lowest): _____

	Optional: 1 cup of herb laxative tea in a.m.	32 oz. water with 2 tsps non-iodized sea salt	No. of 10-ounce lemonade drinks (6 – 12)	Evening 1 cup of herb laxative tea	Comments (wins or detox symptoms)
Night before	N/A	N/A	N/A		
Day 1					
Day 2					
Day 3					
Day 4					
Day 5					
Day 6					
Day 7					
Day 8					
Day 9					
Day 10					

Date Finished: _____ Weight: _____

Measurements: Chest: _____ Waist: _____ Hips: _____ Thighs: _____

Energy level on a scale of one to ten (one being the lowest): _____

Part IV

The Master Cleanse
Discussion Bulletin Board

For those not familiar with an Internet bulletin board, it is a discussion group organized much like a public bulletin board where anyone is free to post their comments for all to see and others are free to post responses to those already posted or to start another topic. Because it is on the Internet, you can see the responses as soon as someone posts them. This allows people to give immediate feedback, to answer questions and to give support for one another, which is what occurs daily on The Master Cleanse Bulletin Board.

I invite you to go to www.TheMasterCleanse.com and click on the bulletin board link to see how this works for yourself.

In this last section, I have used the postings from the month of January 2004 as 110 people did the Master Cleanse on the Internet, plus ten more who weren't on the Internet. I have altered the names of the people writing these comments to provide privacy. I have kept them consistent, so you can see who said what. I have compiled these comments within the topics to which they applied and tried to keep them in date order. The topics have been alphabetized for your convenience.

As far as content, I have had to take some editorial license to edit the topics and postings within them. This is for the most part because of sheer volume. If I had not, this book would be nearly twice as long without adding any new ideas. I have tried to give you an idea of what this bulletin board is like. Hopefully, you will see the feeling of community and support it creates.

After the Cleanse

Peter

After you are done with the cleanse, your body naturally will be inclined to eat raw fruits and vegetables. So, be sure to check out the recipes page at www.TheRawFoodSite.com.

Person No. 1

I am amazed at how my body/mind only wants to consume raw fruits and veggies. Although I have gained three of the fourteen pounds back, I still am one pant size smaller than I was before starting the MC. This statement may be a little far fetched to say but I believe that once the body has gotten rid of toxins, it instinctively craves the fresh, live foods that it so desperately needs to sustain itself and to heal itself. After all, humans have the teeth of herbivores not carnivores.

Person No. 2

I'm on Day 10. Had my one orange for ten minutes, just sat and chewed. Felt very good. I am going to try juicing for another week, then go to raw food. Thanks for all the support and information along the way. A person can't do these things without others. May God bless all of you for your help.

Person No. 3

I am on Day 12 and felt it would emotionally serve me to stop at this point. My tongue was covered with white fuzzy stuff and then when I brushed my teeth, it was completely pink.

I have been reading that after the cleanse I will want to eat fruits and veggies. However, I feel inclined to go towards my old favorites, meat and dairy. Is that a sign that something is wrong or I did it wrong? Also, I was wondering what you know about salt flushing once or twice a week after the cleanse.

Peter

If you did the cleanse and you felt better, you didn't do it wrong. If you're inclined to meat and dairy, that's fine. Try to include some fresh, raw vegetables and fruit in your daily diet as well.

You can always do another cleanse. A fellow I once met told me he'd done the cleanse three times. After the first, he was no longer interested in red meat. After the second cleanse, he found he liked raw vegetables more. After the third, he was no longer interested in meat and wanted organic vegetables. That covered about three years of his life.

My wife and I use salt water flushing whenever we feel we need to wash out our digestive tract after an occasional dinner out with friends. It works great. A healthy diet is a lifelong process, not a one time event.

Person No. 3

Thanks for the quick response. The cleanse was great and I feel so much better. I was wondering what juicing meant. I have read that a few people juice for a week or so after the cleanse. Is that orange juice, grapefruit, or lemonade?

Also, I have found that I love the way I look and feel. How can I prevent my weight coming back? I lost eighteen pounds. I know that diet and food play an important part but is there anything else? This bulletin board has been a life saver. Thanks so much!!!

Peter

Juicing can include a pure juice fast, drinking occasional vegetable juices to rebuild the body, drinking occasional fruit juices to cleanse the body, and everything in between. When I finish a cleanse, I find I want vegetable and fruit juices along with other fresh, raw vegetables, fruit, nuts, and seeds. Others may want nothing but juices for a few days. It's all a matter of what your body wants.

To prevent weight coming back, be sure you eat at least 50% fresh raw vegetables and fruit and if you do eat meat and/or dairy, do a salt water flush the next day. Exercise will also help get your metabolism going to burn calories and to move the fluids in your body. In addition to all this, I recommend doing the Master Cleanse when you feel you need a boost—at least twice a year.

Person No. 67

I appreciate all your time and input. I am now off the cleanse and started with orange juice and have moved into veggies. I am going slow so I can incorporate more fruit and veggies in my diet. However, I am experiencing gas. Is this common and what can I do about it?

Peter

I haven't run into that after the cleanse. I did experience gas the first time I did the cleanse around Day 4. I thought it was gas from the old waste being dissolved by the lemonade. It went away after a couple days.

Burroughs says if you have gas you should continue the cleanse for "several more days."

! Anti-depressants

Person No. 4
After getting everyone else started on this, I am finally ready to do it. I had to wean myself off anti-depressant medication first. It took two weeks.

Peter
Congratulations on getting yourself off the anti-depressant. I recommend the book *Potatoes, not Prozac* by Kathleen DesMaisons (available at www.TheMasterCleanse.com). It points out how a bad diet creates mental distress and a good diet creates a happy, positive mental outlook.

Appendectomy, Recent and Starting a Second Cleanse

Person No. 5
I did the diet for ten days (Dec. 14–24). Not a good time of the year with parties, but I did it. Anyway, I had to have my appendix out a week and one-half ago and was wondering when would be a good time to start another fast? Does the surgery matter? Thanks!

Peter
Ask your surgeon by what date he expects you to be healed completely. Then there will be no question about whether you are getting enough protein to heal the operation scar while you are on the cleanse.

Bentonite and Psyllium During the Cleanse

Person No. 6
Hi, all. I recently read about doing several Bentonite and Psyllium Husk shakes per day with a cleanse. Supposedly it helps with bowel movements and removing mucus layers in the intestine. Has anyone

else heard of this or used this method along with the Master Cleanse? All responses are welcome! Thanks a bunch.

Person No. 7

I've never tried them during this particular cleanse but I have used them with other cleanses (juicing and such) and had good results. After I finished this cleanse (two days ago) and started eating whole foods again I introduced psyllium and organic ground flax seeds in my diet to help my colon get back into shape. If you're going to do this, drink plenty of water before and afterward since it absorbs lots of it once it's down. Personally, I find that using the senna tea for a long period of time is like trying to run five miles after not wearing your shoes for a few months.

It's probably best to stick to the program to get the best results. However, I would like to hear from others who have done this during the cleanse and hear their results.

Person No. 8

From what I have read, it is not good to stay on senna tea for long term because it irritates your colon. That is why it works for the cleanse. Psyllium husk is not good to be on because it robs your colon of water and the most important thing you need for good bowel movements is at least eight glasses a day. I am reading a book right now called *Your Body's Many Cries for Water*. The author (F. Batmanghelidj, M.D.) states that all diseases can be cured if the body has sufficient water. A lot of the stuff he says makes sense. So even though I go to the bathroom a lot anyway, I am trying to drink eight glasses of water a day.

Person No. 9

In doing research about the Master Cleanse, I found a website that talks about "The Ultimate Fast." It sounds like the Master Cleanse except that certain products are added: one for parasites, something called a Colon Cleanse tablet, and psyllium and bentonite products. It has links to buy the products, too. It goes for eight days and then with modifications for ninety days.

I was just wondering if anyone knew if these steps were really necessary for complete and thorough cleansing, including the elimination of parasites. I thought psyllium was a form of fiber, although I could be wrong, but if I'm not, that means your colon really wouldn't be "resting" throughout the cleanse, right? I am interested in the bentonite thing, because the website I found claims it's the only thing known to remove plaque from the walls of the intestines and colon. Having Crohn's disease, I think that would be especially beneficial.

I'm doing my shopping for the cleanse tomorrow and wasn't sure if I needed this added stuff. I'm excited! Thank you again.

Person No. 8
Sounds to me like they are trying to sell you their products that you don't need. Just follow the Master Cleanse as written and it will get rid of the toxins and gunk in your body.

Person No. 9
That's what I figured, too. I'm still going to research that bentonite stuff, though. I'm curious now! Thanks.

Person No. 8
Yeah, the bentonite sounds interesting since they say that is the only thing that will remove the plaque from the walls of the intestines. I checked the site more thoroughly and they also promote the Awareness products which I used when I started the Hallelujah Diet. They are very expensive and really not necessary. You can do more with the Master Cleanse and eating raw fruits, vegetables, nuts and seeds when you are done. However, I wonder if the bentonite will clean more of the mucus buildup so someone doesn't need to do a twenty-day cleanse to really get rid of stuff. My husband just did twenty days (I only made it six) and he probably wouldn't go twenty days again.

Peter
After I did my first twenty-day cleanse a year ago, I decided to do the Schultz herbal cleanse with herbs, psyllium and bentonite clay. I did it for ten days and didn't think it did anything for me as I was already quite clean from the Master Cleanse.

As to whether the bentonite clay is the only way to remove old waste on the colon walls, I go by the appearance of the tongue. (Chinese doctors have used the tongue to diagnose internal organs for thousands of years and I'm amazed at what it reveals during the cleanse! Check the topic "Tongue Coating" below for more info.) When I check tongue color, I've discovered that the two people I know who have eaten a pure raw veggie, fruit, nut and seed diet have perfectly pink tongues, just like Burroughs says. I've also produced a perfectly pink tongue after a seventeen-day cleanse and seven days of adding one ounce of wheatgrass juice to my raw food diet. Based on that, I would say that the bentonite clay is not the only way to remove old waste on the colon walls and that psyllium is not necessary either. I agree it's better to let the colon and body take a rest from digestion in order to detox.

Boredom

Person No. 6
One acute symptom I am feeling during this fast is boredom now that I taken myself off eating, I'm experiencing a peaceful sort of tiredness where I don't feel like doing much of anything. This is Day 1 of my cleanse. I figure this must be one of those uncomfortable times in life where you feel alone, when in truth you really are not. So, besides reading and watching TV, what are people doing when they're bored and really want to eat something solid? How do you keep your mind preoccupied with anything other than food? Any input would be greatly appreciated. Thanks!

Person No. 11
I went to Google [www.Google.com, a search website on the Internet] and typed in "I am bored" and hit the search button! Ok, that was when I was desperate! Aside from that, I read. It makes time fly. Or I paint, or I practice my bass, or I go take a little catnap. Mainly I have been Googling "Master Cleanse" to find out as much as I can about people's experience on this fast. Oh, and I can't forget, I spend a lot of time trying to get my friends to do this with me! Then we can all whine to each other and I wouldn't feel so alone. Finding this site helped a lot though. I think I will probably do some Pilates today. Not for boredom but to give my body some much needed exercise! Good luck with the cleanse, stick with it! I'm on Day 4 and I am already feeling great! I can only imagine Day 10!

Person No. 6
Thanks for responding to this topic! I thought maybe I was the only one losing my mind over this thing! This is Day 2 for me and I can honestly say that I feel good. The bored-out-of-my-skull, listless feelings I had yesterday, are not present right now. I don't feel lethargic. I can

move again! And my mind isn't totally on food today! So Day 2 is definitely better for me than Day 1. Oh, by the way, as far as being bored is concerned, I think I also drove Google crazy typing in any word in relation to the Master Cleanse that I thought might help me along, i.e. "Master Cleanse journey," "Master Cleanse journal," etc. To combat boredom I started a journal, wrote a ton of poetry, laughed out loud at mindless sitcoms, fell asleep on a really good novel a couple of times, and, of course, prayer and more prayer.

Person No. 11

That's wonderful! It's great that you are keeping an upbeat attitude! Just think of all the good this is doing to your body! Last night I had a very emotional AND spiritual detox experience. I pray every night before bed of course, but last night was different. I was emotionally overcome and I cried and cried, not because I was sad. I think it was because so much clutter is being removed from my body and my mind. It's hard to explain accurately but suffice it to say, that I felt like a weight had been lifted off my shoulders when I was done. I dedicated my ten-day fast to God, so it makes it a little easier to resist the temptation to give in. I just think of all He has given me — ten days is nothing in comparison! Anyway, best of luck to you on this cleanse! Update me on any other ways you are combating boredom!

Peter

It sounds like you two are doing great on the cleanse. I would like to add that boredom or being listless is just another detox symptom.

Person No. 12

What great wonderful things I just read in this topic! I just want to say that I had a dream I kicked a soccer ball in the goal. This may not sound important to you, but as a child of elementary age I played soccer and was not ever really good. I am glad I played soccer because I believe sports are wonderful for young children and I think being good at sports has to do with practice as well as being in a confident mindset.

Anyway I kept having these recurring dreams that disturbed me for many years of adulthood. The dreams were of me playing soccer as a child and never getting the ball in the goal. I would miss the ball or mess up, feeling frustrated when I woke up.

So, this dream of succeeding at getting the ball in the goal was an accomplishment I've desired. Though I may never be a great soccer player physically, the dream was enough to satisfy my subconscious mind.

Thank you for your postings. I feel great and look forward to a detox of my body—and mind as well!

Bowel Movements

Person No. 13
Is everyone here using organic lemons? I had some conventional lemons left from before I started my fast, which never seemed to give me problems. So, that is what I have been using. But I am starting to think this is part of what is making this cleanse so painful for me. My butt is on fire when I eliminate now. I'm wondering if the chemicals in the conventional lemons are just too harsh on an empty stomach like this. Tomorrow I will get some organics.

Peter
The burning poops are caused by the toxins leaving your body. Toxins are acid. They burn. The first cleanse I did was so bad I had to put some vitamin E on my butt for Days 2–5. By then, the burning stopped and only came back on the seventh day.

Person No. 13
Thanks for your reply. I guess I'll just have to deal with the burning, but I am going to switch to organic lemons anyway. No point in putting more chemicals back in my body while I'm trying to get them out to begin with.

Person No. 1
Now that you mention hot poop—before I completed the ten-day MC, I did a thirty-six-hour MC because I had never fasted before. Afterwards, I felt really great and ate raw fruit and veggies and fresh juice for five days. Then I started the ten-day MC. It was the evening of Day 1 of the ten-day MC that I had a really hot BM. I thought I was literally eliminating hot flames from my butt. It was much hotter than a burning sensation. Then I did some research and found out that my body was probably eliminating acid toxins. WOW!

Person No. 14

Just wanted to clarify something. I usually have a BM on awakening which I presume is from the laxative tea. I then drink the SWF (salt water flush) and within an hour I have as many as five BMs. Should I be having more BMs throughout the day? I am not, but reading other people's experiences, they seem to have far more eliminations. Am I doing it right? I would be grateful for any thoughts on this and experiences that anyone else is having. Thanks a lot.

Person No. 15

I'm having the exact same problem, only worse. I'm on my third day and am not having any BMs throughout the day. I haven't from the beginning. I'm only having the kind that are runny or just yellow liquid in the morning—pretty gross. Plus, the laxative tea is giving me severe cramps in the middle of the night. The back of the package says you should stop taking it if you find there's discomfort, so I don't know what to do. I'm following the directions exactly. What I want to know is, will this change? I don't think I should go for ten days if this persists.

● Peter

Here is my experience with four Master Cleanses over the last year. For the first few days of the first cleanse, I had only one semi-solid BM in the morning. After a few days, I'd have one very watery BM first thing in the morning and then several (four or so) watery flushes from the salt water starting thirty to sixty minutes after drinking it and lasting for an hour or two. I had no more BMs after that for the rest of the day. After Day 10 on the first fast (it was a twenty-day fast), I might have had one or two more small, very watery BMs during the rest of the day.

On later cleanses, I would have more watery flushes after only two or three days, but none after that during the day. The watery ones are always bright yellow. Usually there are small brown mucousy flakes that I believe are the broken down remains of older waste.

Runny BMs are the norm on the cleanse. Solid ones are unusual after the first day, although my last cleanse had semi-solid ones for the first seven days. It would mean very old layers coming off the colon walls. Normally, these older layers are dissolved by the cayenne and lemon juice and that's why they are not solid. In my case, the solid

47

ones were accompanied by major detox symptoms the day before and feeling even better after the BM.

Concerning abdominal cramps from the laxative tea, when you get past Day 5 or so, due to less waste in the intestines, you can feel the intestinal contractions. At times, they are uncomfortable.

They can be handled by:

1) Using an herbal tea that is a combination rather than pure senna tea;

2) Drinking water or lemonade to give the intestines something to push along rather than just cramp up the muscles; and

3) Reducing the amount of tea to half a cup and then filling it with water so that it is diluted by half.

These contractions are occasional for me and when they are present they are uncomfortable, but not painful, except for one or two days when they were painful for perhaps fifteen minutes before I went to the bathroom. Then the cramps disappeared completely.

If yours are truly painful and last more than two days and the above three things don't handle, then you should probably discontinue the herbal laxative tea. However, then you MUST be doing the salt water as I do NOT recommend anyone do this cleanse without elimination aids. There are just too many toxins released.

Person No. 14

Peter, thanks for such reassuring information. Instinctively I felt what I was experiencing was right but when you start reading other people's posts, the doubts creep in. Your experiences with the cleanse pretty much mirror my own. I now feel okay. I'm just starting Day 5. I have only had minimal weight loss but my body feels a lot different. (I was near to my ideal weight any way.) I woke up at 6:30 (with a little bit of help from two small kids) and didn't feel at all groggy. Wow, that is a new experience for me. Overall I am feeling just great. I'm not finding the Master Cleanse a picnic by any means (I'm really craving fruit and veggies) but it is so doable and I am loving the results. Thanks so much to all for your advice and encouragement.

Person No. 15

Sounds like you are doing great on the MC, too. I guess logically there wouldn't be much bowel activity through the day as you eliminate most of it with the flush. Also, I guess the word "flush" suggests something fast and complete. I suppose reading other people's comments can be good if it backs up what you are experiencing, but it can cast doubts when it doesn't. I think you and I are doing just great and probably having textbook reactions. Perhaps, we both need to have more faith in our bodies to do the right thing. I know I do. Good luck with the rest of the cleanse.

Person No. 12

Ok, I've been reading and reading all these comments, questions and responses. I am a little confused on the bowel movements. I am on Day 4 today and my bowel movement (diarrhea-like liquid) is early in the morning. After that, I drink the salt water and then my movement is completely water, the color of lemonade.

In some responses, it says the solid bowel movements may come around Day 8-10 according to the person's body and toxins. However, in others it says if you continue to have diarrhea after Day 4 or 5, you should seek a doctor and stop the cleanse.

I have not had a solid movement since I started this cleanse! I went on this diet after coming off the Atkins diet for about a week or so. So, I think I am really stopped up with cheese and meat!

Also my diet has been bad for a long time and I worked in a bar for many years and drank alcohol regularly and smoked when I drank. I know I have lots of toxins to be released. Is the one-time morning movement of diarrhea-like liquid followed by the water release normal?? I know the tea is causing my early diarrhea-like bowel movement and the salt water is causing the flush, but is there hope for a solid movement? How long should I wait?

Person No. 13

I can't speak from experience much, since this is my first time doing the cleanse, but if you are just coming off Atkins you are VERY stopped up. I did Atkins a couple of years ago and I was constantly constipated. I am probably still getting rid of stuff from back then, or will be during this cleanse.

I'm sure the moderator will reply, and you should listen to what he says above all, because he's done this cleanse many times. But I would say, if you feel okay, keep it up till you get a solid movement. That one movement of diarrhea per day is probably not enough to harm you as long as you are drinking enough fluids to replace what you lose— and on this cleanse you should be. I think you will eventually see results. It's just going to take some time for that impacted stuff to break apart and come out.

Person No. 12

Thanks. I appreciate the response. I was beginning to get worried. I have been a little constipated from Atkins so I will wait it out. Other than that, I feel fine. I am cold a lot with chills and a little stuffy. That's about it. My energy has not really increased much, but my mornings are definitely NOT groggy! I am sooo looking forward to the brighter days ahead. I have had some very strange dreams—dreams that I am conquering a fear I had since I was kid!! I think that is a definite enlightenment from this diet! I hope you are doing well too. I have read your postings. Good luck.

Person No. 1

Hang in there. Day 2 through 4, I had flu-like symptoms. I had liquid, mucousy movements as you described. Then on Day 6, I eliminated some intestinal-shaped matter about three to four feet long. No more really extensive toilet inspections for me after that! It was pretty scary. Then, I had a few more days of liquid, mucousy movements. Later on Days 8, 9 and 10, I eliminated stuff that smelled like the real thing. (So, I guess it was the real thing.) After that, I extended my cleanse beyond the minimum ten-day recommendation.

I have read that the intestines detox in layers. So your intestines will remove any old, built-up layers over time. Therefore you will have periods of liquid and mucousy BMs and then mucousy and solid BMs. Based on my experience this is true. Therefore it is very important to drink the correct lemonade formula, use the salt water cleanse in the mornings and laxative tea at night before bed and drink additional water during the day as well.

Every person's body is not the same. Hang in there and do not quit! Your body is just detoxing.

Good luck to you all! I'll be back the last week in March.

Person No. 12
Thanks to you all. Cool deal! I feel better now. Can't wait to pass the mass!

Person No. 11
I am on Day 9 and I have yet to have any solid BMs. Mine are all runny. However, they're not only liquid. There is stuff in there that needed to get out. I am wondering if I will have any solid BMs at all! If I don't, is that bad? Also, it is not recommended to drink senna tea for more than seven days. Any suggestions? I just can't keep the salt water down, even with warm water.

Peter
Re: Runny vs. solid BMs. All the others have been quite correct in their postings. The waste of a lifetime comes off in layers and takes quite a while to dissolve if you've been eating a diet heavy in meat and dairy. But don't worry, the lemonade WILL dissolve it.

[There is more about senna tea in the "Laxative tea" topic below.]

Person No. 12
Thank you, Peter, for your time, energy and advice. You are making a world of a difference in my life and many others! We all appreciate it.

Person No. 13
When I eliminate, the liquid that comes out has consistently been a neon yellow color so far. Is this acid or bile and are other people having this happen? (I know acid is coming out. I wasn't sure if that is what contributed to the color though.)

Peter
To my knowledge, it always happens. I believe the yellow is from bile. Does anyone have any other data on this?

Person No. 16
It's from the vitamin Bs in the maple syrup. Vitamin B_6 and sometimes B_{12} causes your pee to be highlighter yellow.

Person No. 13
Ah, danke (thank you).

Person No. 17

It is true that B vitamins cause your pee to be yellow, but I think we are referring to the yellow color of our BM liquid. I tend to agree with Peter that it is the bile or perhaps the lemonade?

Peter

Probably bile, rather than lemonade. There's just not enough yellow color in the lemons.

It is true that B_{12} and other B vitamins turn your pee yellow, but I've never seen them turn my BMs yellow.

Person No. 12

My BMs have gotten darker and darker as the days have gone by. I am happy with that. They have a little more texture, but still liquid. Gosh, I haven't had one thing solid to eat in ten days and it's still flowing out. Amazing! How funny to chat about our private pooping experiences. I love it!

Person No. 18

I'm on Day 7 and I'm still amazed too. Mine also gets darker and darker each day. I guess the deeper the "do," the darker the hue. Okay, that's the lemonade talking. Not only is it funny to be talking about our bowel movements, but I think I've become borderline obsessive about them. Can't read enough of this stuff.

Person No. 13

Yeah, I'm obsessive too. My favorite part is looking in the toilet to see what came out each time. It makes the pain I go through (that tea makes me hurt) worth it. Boy, I am not pleased to know what was in me all that time, but I am so pleased to see it come out.

Mine is not getting darker and darker like that, though. It was really dark the first couple days. Now I am just getting these little bits and pieces of things (mostly old rotten meat—yuck!). Maybe I got the big initial stuff out and now I am just chipping away at the rest. That is what I hope. Today is Day 8. I haven't had a big mass come out since Day 2.

Bowel Movements Not Happening

Person No. 19

Hi. Today is my third day on the cleanse, and I haven't had a BM since Day 1. Because I didn't go yesterday, I increased my salt to three teaspoons today, but it still didn't work. Any suggestions? Thanks.

Peter

Just ensure you are doing the laxative tea at night and the salt water flush in the morning and six to twelve drinks of lemonade with fresh lemon juice as instructed in the book. Then if you still are not eliminating, add a single cup of laxative tea first thing in the morning as well. Beyond that, don't worry. The cleanse will work it out, believe me.

Some people come to the Master Cleanse from the Atkins diet and have eaten heavily of dairy and meat and white flour products. Worse, they may have been taking medicines and many of them are constipated as a side effect. Sometimes it takes a few days.

Person No. 16

I'm in the beginning of Day 3 and I've only made one bowel movement on Day 1. This morning I drank half a quart of the salt water flush. I couldn't muster it all. I did the herbal tea last night. Why isn't there any elimination?

Peter

1. People who eat SAD (the Standard American Diet of meat, dairy, 100% cooked food, no raw vegetables, very few if any raw fruits) get "plugged up" and it can take two or three days before the full quart salt water flush begins to eliminate.

2. Not drinking at least six ten-ounce drinks of lemonade a day (or more for larger people) makes for less eliminations.

3. The salt water flush not only produces several liquid eliminations starting within thirty to sixty minutes, but also provides liquid in the colon to promote and make later eliminations easier.

So, 1) be patient, 2) drink lots of lemonade, and 3) do the salt water flush when at all possible.

By the way, some people think if they eliminate only a bright yellow liquid that it doesn't count as a bowel movement. I consider anything that comes out the "back end" as a bowel movement.

Person No. 20

Hi. This is the first time I have tried the MC. I am in Day 3 and I am having a bit of a problem. I am not hungry or anything but I am not having any BMs. Yesterday I had a small one but that's it. I am not taking the salt water because it makes me vomit, but I am drinking the laxative tea. What can I do?

Person No. 21

I'm a newbie too, but I'm on Day 10. I've read that if you can't tolerate the salt water flush that you can do the laxative tea morning and night. Also you need to be sure you're drinking enough water in addition to the lemonade. I usually alternate water with the lemonade. That should help move things along. When you tried the salt water flush did you use pure sea salt with no additives? It is much easier to tolerate than regular salt. I had been using sea salt, but I noticed after reading more closely that it had non-clumping agents. I bought some without that and it is much easier to drink. I drink it with a straw really quickly so I don't have to really taste it. The first time I did it I nearly threw up, but now I'm used to it, especially since I've been using the straw.

Person No. 20

Thanks. I think that the problem is that I am not drinking enough water. I did use sea salt—the only kind that was available to me from a health food store. I am going to try to drink more water.

Peter

Be sure you are mixing your lemonade according to the book and drinking at least six to twelve glasses per day, drinking the quart of salt water (with two level teaspoons of sea salt) first thing in the morning and laxative tea (I recommend a blend with senna in it, not straight senna) morning and evening until you are eliminating more.

Person No. 3

I am on Day 4 and still have a sinus infection. I am starting to have some BMs but not much. I am going back to my herbal colon cleanse. The tea did nothing for me. I really am tired. My spirits are high and I feel pretty good all around. However, I know that my real detox hasn't started yet.

Peter

I'm sorry to hear that you needed to go back to your herbal colon cleanse. For the sake of my education on the cleanse, can you answer a few questions to help me know exactly where it went wrong for you?

Can you tell me exactly how you had been mixing your lemonade?

How much of it you were drinking per day?

How you mixed your salt water?

Did you do it (salt water flush) every day?

What herbal laxative tea you used?

Did you drink it every night?

Did you take or eat anything else while on the cleanse?

What was your diet like before the cleanse?

Do you take any medications? (You don't need to be specific as to which ones.)

How long have you been taking the herbal colon cleanse?

[Unfortunately, Person No. 3 never answered the questions.]

● Breaking the Fast—Very Important

Peter

Breaking a long fast correctly is very, very important. If you go right to solid food, devouring everything in sight, you're going to feel very sick to your stomach or worse... much worse. You should ease your way back to solid food by following the instructions on breaking the fast. Burroughs says drink fresh-squeezed orange juice, but I found that too heavy at times and so substituted fresh grapefruit juice.

If you are going to be eating raw fruits and vegetables, you may eat raw fruit for lunch on the third day with a raw salad for dinner. (Many people naturally gravitate to healthier raw vegetables, fruits and juices to preserve the good feelings they gained on the cleanse.)

If you have been a meat and/or milk products consumer, shift to homemade (not canned or packaged) vegetable soup for dinner the second day. Have orange juice for breakfast the third day with the vegetable soup for lunch and a salad for dinner. Keep the Master Cleanse lemonade drink as your breakfast drink after that. You will do better with less meat and no milk products as they are very productive of mucus and hinder digestion and absorption of nutrients. (Also see pages 25–27 of *The Master Cleanser* for Burroughs' details on breaking the fast.)

Person No. 16

I was going really strong. Today would be my ninth day. I had laxative tea this morning, intending to go forth with my cleanse, maybe even for another week, but I was really hungry when I went to the store to get more syrup and my mom and I bought a lot of fruits for me to dehydrate and eat when I went off the cleanse. (I was going to finish in two days.) However, when I got home I was very hungry and wanted fruit so badly that, even before having orange juice, I had a few green grapes, a few glasses of orange juice, and a bite of apple I was cutting to dehydrate it. I thought it would be okay since I had been on the cleanse, perfectly, for eight days, but my stomach is hurting now even though I've had a lot of water to try to make the stomachache go away. What do I do?

Peter

I've done the exact same thing although it was after ten days. I drank orange juice, ate an orange, a salad, then some almonds, pepperoncini, olives, etc. Within thirty to forty-five minutes, I was sorry because I had nausea and an upset stomach. It lasted through the afternoon, but went away gradually that evening.

In my personal experience, the discomfort of breaking the fast the wrong way (eating solid foods too soon) goes away after a day or less. I have heard a second-hand story that I have not been able to verify that much more serious medical consequences are possible if you break your fast without a gradual return to "normal" food.

Person No. 22

Peter, what was wrong with what you ate? Was it that you rushed into a variety of solid foods, or that you just rushed into solid foods period?

Also, someone mentioned earlier that returning to a solid food diet will cause lost weight to return. Is this true? Thanks.

Peter

It was that I rushed into solid foods too fast.

As far as solid food causing weight to return, I eat solid food and after two years weigh the same or less than after my first Master Cleanse. It is what you eat. Toxins, preservatives, chemicals your body cannot digest will put on the weight because your body protects itself by putting those toxins in fat cells.

Person No. 14

I am planning on stopping after Day 10. Do you stop everything that you have been having on the fast and just start purely on the juice? How much juice do you drink? Is it breakfast, lunch and dinner or whenever you feel hungry? Can you give me a rough estimate of how many oranges I should be juicing? Can I mix it up a bit and have some grapefruit juice and some orange juice? Many thanks for your help.

Peter

Burroughs says to slowly drink several eight-ounce glasses of fresh orange juice the first two days—with extra water if you want.
He goes on to recommend eating vegetable soup in the evening. I have personally found the orange juice too "thick," almost like eating solid food, and instead used grapefruit juice.

My own experience, having done solid food the first day afterwards and being nauseated, is that you need to be on just juices or you'll feel nauseated. I know of one person who vomited because she went back to solid food the next day.

Brushing Your Teeth During the Cleanse

Peter

I've had several people ask about brushing their teeth on the cleanse. Burroughs makes no comments one way or another. I see no reason not to brush your teeth. I do it with just water, but I don't know of any problem using salt, if you want to do that. What have others done?

Person No. 23

I use IPSAB brand tooth powder. It's a combo of salt, baking soda, prickly ash bark and peppermint oil. It doesn't have all the fillers and other stuff in traditional toothpaste. It also works great on the film on your tongue. I bought it at a health food store.

Candida

Person No. 24

Any feedback on yeast and the MC? Does the maple syrup feed the yeast? Is the cleanse effective for yeast buildup as well as others kinds of toxins? My husband is considering joining us but is concerned about the yeast factor. Thanks. Love and light to all.

Peter

I'm aware of the conventional medical thought that yeast is caused by sugar and therefore all sweets should be avoided. I'm also aware that this (avoiding sweets) doesn't seem more than a "Band-Aid" for sufferers and I've heard no miracle cures.

I'm also aware of Victoria Boutenko, a raw food author (*The Raw Family* and *12 Steps to Raw Food*) and lecturer, who has a different perception on handling yeast. She says it can be handled by eliminating all fats and oils from the diet for a period of time. You see, fat metabolism and sugar metabolism are linked. You cannot digest sugar without fat! Some even say diabetes is actually the result of a failure of the body to handle fat.

Per Victoria, it takes from three days to two weeks depending on how severe the yeast infection is. That is also about the length of the Master Cleanse. Perhaps that is the reason that I have never heard anyone complain about yeast on the Master Cleanse.

Person No. 17

My mom has systemic yeast problems and did the cleanse for thirty days. It helped her a lot, but I am afraid I don't have a lot of details about her experience.

Person No. 12

I don't have bad problems with yeast but I have had in the past. I notice it when my diet goes downhill. I have not had any problem with yeast on this fast.

● Cayenne Pepper

Peter

Cayenne pepper is such a wonderful herb. I want to share a great web page explaining its virtues. Some people wonder what it does in the Master Cleanse. Here's a good link for more information: www.shirleys-wellness-cafe.com/cayenne.htm.

Person No. 2

OK, I believe you. I am back to putting cayenne pepper in the lemonade. Took Day 4 off from the pepper. Good article, and a must read for anyone making lemonade.

Person No. 16

I don't have any cayenne pepper at the moment. I started the cleanse today. If I don't use the pepper for the first few days, will that affect the results of the cleanse?

Person No. 1

The pepper is very important. Check out the first posting at the top of this topic and go buy the pepper.

If you want great results, don't alter the directions in any way for the cleanse. If you do not have a copy of the Master Cleanse book, buy one. Follow the directions and Good luck!

Person No. 6

I like to use a lot of cayenne pepper. Love the taste. But will overdoing the cayenne alter results? I like to use about 1/2 tsp. per glass. My lemonade is pretty red. Does anyone else out there overdose on the cayenne? If so, what were the results? By the way, everything else is measured out to the T. And I make it two glasses at a time, because one glass doesn't usually satisfy me.

Peter

In *The Master Cleanser*, Stanley Burroughs says to use a tenth of a teaspoon of cayenne or "to taste." So, add all you want. Like you, my son loves it, put in much more than 1/10th teaspoon and had a great result.

Person No. 25

I'm just wondering whether it's okay to take cayenne tablets instead of putting it in the lemon drink.

Peter

Do not take cayenne in capsules.

According to Dr. Schulze, a master herbalist, people who take cayenne capsules do not receive much of the benefit of the cayenne. The nerve endings in the mouth respond almost instantly to send blood throughout the body. This whole process is missed if you take capsules. Furthermore, gelatin is made from boiled skin, bones and tendons. That is a lot of digestive work — especially when you are not eating food to give your digestive system a chance to cleanse itself. So, taking cayenne capsules should not be done.

If you "can't drink cayenne" it is usually because you took too much at some time before this. Start with just a sprinkle and gradually increase it as you tolerate more. Decide to learn to take cayenne. It is wonderful for your health.

Here is a link to a great web page on cayenne: http://www.herbsfirst.com/NewsLetters/0299cayenne.html

As a side note, there are three things that will make cayenne hotter: 1) Mixing up a whole day's batch and putting cayenne in the drink when you make it. This is because cayenne gets stronger the longer it sits in the drink. 2) Not shaking or stirring the container before drinking. This is especially true if you work and mix several glasses at once. The cayenne will sink to the bottom and the last sips will be very, very hot. 3) There are several strengths of cayenne. The common one sold in supermarkets is usually 30,000 heat units. Health food stores usually carry that kind and an African Bird cayenne that is more than twice as hot!

Cheating—Am I Alone?

Person No. 26

Well, I blew it. I ate an orange Sunday morning and ate salad, nuts and olives at a birthday party last night. I feel really bad. I was working very hard, there were a lot of detox symptoms, and I really wanted to get through ten days at least, though I suspect I need more. Anyway, I plan on eating better and trying again in April. Do you have any thoughts? I could sure use some guidance.

Peter

I'm assuming that you blew it after only two or three days or close to the seventh day as usually those are the ones where the cravings and detox are the worst.

Don't beat yourself up! You took a step forward and did something good for your body. Take pride in the initial step.

You didn't give details, but the first thing I'd check is whether you followed the directions in the book exactly. Herbal laxative tea at night, salt water flush every morning, six to twelve ten-ounce drinks of lemonade in the right proportions each day, and nothing else except water and perhaps mint tea? If you deviated, you'll make it tough on yourself as you'll not be eliminating the toxins you're mobilizing and they'll just reabsorb and you'll have heavy detox symptoms. If that was the case, it was wise that you went off what you thought was "the cleanse."

Have you a serious caffeine habit—sodas, coffee or even a heavy tea habit? If so, it may take a while to break it. (See the topic "Quitting Smoking at the Same Time" below. It is about addictions. It will give you hope.)

Think of cleansing and diet as a lifelong process, not as a one-time event. You don't get a cleansing report card and then go on to other things in life. You learn about you and your body and how the two of you need to get along. Work toward eating more raw vegetables, fruits, nuts, and seeds. Have some fresh juices. Do the Master Cleanse again. I hope this helps.

The urgent desire to eat something else, anything else, and the desire just to CHEW something are both detox symptoms that will pass with the next elimination or two.

Someone mentioned a metallic taste in the mouth. That is also a detox symptom and probably a sign that person has a greater than average amount of toxins to eliminate. In cases such as this, sometimes the full ten days are needed to get the best results.

Person No. 27

Well, I was doing well, but then Day 3 hit, and it was HORRIBLE—just hungry all day, and a massive headache. No specific cravings, just intense hunger no matter how much lemonade I had.

I made it through Day 3, but then on Day 4 (yesterday) I caved, and ate a big piece of bread, which I promptly threw up quite violently within fifteen minutes! They are not kidding when they say you have to ease back into eating. Then I hated myself, felt really sick and had diarrhea for the next five hours or so, so I don't think I absorbed much of the bread! By the evening I felt better and went back on the lemonade.

I decided to just stick with the fast, and am on Day 5 now, feeling great. Or should I really be calling this Day 1, since I cheated yesterday? Come on, 'fess up, has anyone else caved on the cleanse and then continued anyway? I feel really good, have lost seven pounds so far, and I don't just want to give up all the benefits now!

Person No. 17

I have had three dreams on three different nights that I ate food and broke my fast. In all the dreams I was so mad at myself for cheating. Thankfully in my waking state I have not allowed a speck of food to part my lips. However, one day I put my daughter's reheated, leftover pizza to my nose and inhaled deeply for about three minutes. Such ecstasy!

Chemotherapy, Cancer and the Cleanse

Person No. 28

I was diagnosed with ovarian cancer two years ago. I did everything to avoid chemo, but I ended up with no choice. I ended my treatment last June and my prognosis is very good. No cancer cells in my blood tests. I am starting the Master Cleanse tomorrow and looking forward to feeling detoxified. I have heard that detoxifying too fast could stir up too many toxins in the lymph system and be dangerous because my lymph system might not be able to handle it. This cleanse sounds like it is more of a digestive cleanse than a lymph cleanse, but I would like your opinion. Have you had others that needed to detoxify from chemo? Thank you

Peter

I'm glad you asked before leaping into the cleanse. Ask your health professional before starting the cleanse as your concern about detoxifying too fast is important. Then, if you decide to do the cleanse and, considering you have had chemo, I would just "stick a toe in the water" and only drink the minimum six drinks of lemonade each day.

I would also be sure to take the herbal laxative tea in the evening and drink at least one ounce of water or lemonade for each two pounds of your body weight each day. Be sure to do the salt water flush as given each morning, and take long, soaking hot baths with Epsom salts to draw out toxins. (*Do not do this in fluoridated water!* Fluoride is more toxic than lead and a serious enzyme inhibitor. Cancer patients and survivors must avoid drinking, bathing or showering in fluoridated water.)

The reason for the above is that with the potential toxins in your body, you want to detoxify very lightly, but use a maximum of elimination methods so that whatever is loosened/mobilized will be quickly eliminated.

Next, I would immediately discontinue the cleanse if any detox symptoms didn't disappear or lessen with the next day's eliminations.

Day 2 and 3 are usually the worst. Day 7 or 8 is usually the next worse. If you are feeling bad on Day 4, I would discontinue the cleanse and eat fresh raw veggies, fruit, nuts and seeds for a month or so. Even then, you may have to eat some cooked rice or bread to slow down the raw food detox depending on symptoms.

You can do the Master Cleanse several times, so don't try to push it.

Person No. 68

In August, I was diagnosed with a brain tumor. Most days are filled with headaches, dizziness, nausea, and some visual/balance problems. I've never had regular bowel movements and have always had bloating, gas, and several problems because of that. Since starting the cleanse, all those symptoms have disappeared and I've lost twelve pounds. I'm completely thrilled!! I go back to the neurologist Monday and can't wait to tell him all this.

I plan to eat much healthier, (after breaking the fast appropriately). I have more energy and clarity and feel more like myself.

I just wanted to give my "testimony." This has been a godsend.

Chewing Gum

Person No. 29

I started the MC today, 5 Jan 2004. It is very encouraging and motivating to read everyone's questions and comments. I am so excited for my own outcome. I do have a question. Can you chew any kind of gum? Thanks.

Peter

No. Chewing gum consists of five main ingredients: a gum base, sugar, corn syrup, softeners, and flavorings. Some gums include artificial chemicals to sweeten them. These have to be handled by the body as toxins.

Other than a cup of herbal laxative tea in the evening (and optionally one in the morning), a quart of (sea) salt water first thing in the morning, six to twelve drinks of lemon (or lime)ade during the day, occasional mint tea and as much water as you want, nothing else is a part of Stanley Burrough's Master Cleanse regimen. The idea is to give the digestive and elimination organs a rest so they can use their energy to cleanse and rejuvenate.

Cleansing, Other Types

Person No. 1
Is it really necessary for people to do a liver cleanse with olive oil after they complete the Master Cleanse? I am a little hesitant. I was under the impression that the MC was cleaning the liver as well as other internal organs.

Peter
You're correct that the Master Cleanse does also cleanse the liver, kidneys, glands and other parts of the body. People with arthritis have even commented that they noticed joint pain relieved or eliminated.

I have a good friend and business partner who did a ten-day cleanse. He has had a massage every week for several years from his massage therapist. The second week of his cleanse, she told him he had the cleanest liver she'd ever observed. She also said she's never seen anyone's body change so much for the better in her professional life.

I'd be very interested in feedback from people that do another kind of cleanse after the Master Cleanse to see if they notice any difference.

Person No. 1
Peter, Thank you so very much for this website!

Your responses to my questions and the feedback from others have been very helpful. This is Day 10 of the MC for me and my tongue is very pink and my breath smells good! I have decided to extend my fast a few more days to see if I will have any additional effects/benefits.

Question: Is it safe to say that with an extended MC fast at some point in time the body will start eliminating all mucus and nothing else?

Peter

Definitely, although the waste does come off in layers.

When I did my first cleanse (twenty days), I had just bright yellow (bile?) liquid after the eighth day. However, on the seventeenth day, I passed some semi-solid waste!

I'm on Day 16 of my third cleanse and for the first ten days, I had some semi-solid material every day. It's quite amazing how much stuff there is inside a person.

Cold, Feeling

Person No. 12

I am cold all day long and all night. I am trying to stay warm. I have turned up the heat, put on more clothes etc. I have been getting the chills ever since I started this cleanse. I sure hope this is a common side effect. The weather here in Atlanta goes up and down, some days colder than others. Even when I'm inside I'm cold. My hands, feet and nose are the coldest! Anyone else?

Person No. 8

Yea, I don't know why Peter couldn't have suggested doing this in July when the chills would feel good! Anyway, the pepper is supposed to help with the chills, so if you can add more pepper it might help. That's one of the reasons I like the capsules, because then I could do more pepper and not feel quite as cold. We also heated up the lemonade one day just because we were so cold. You don't get as much benefit from it but it felt good.

Person No. 13

I was a bit cold my first couple days. Now as of my sixth day I don't seem to be having that problem anymore.

Person No. 6

Today is Day 10 for me! And I have to say that I have had the chills from Day 1 until today. Glad to know it's not just me. But I have been freezing throughout the entire cleanse! Fleece is my friend!

Peter

Any sort of fasting lowers metabolism and that means the body is colder. The Master Cleanse fits right in there.

As for July instead of January, that's a great idea. Actually, I was planning to promote Master Cleanses quarterly, but seeing all the great results people are getting, I think I will just promote cleanses whenever someone is ready.

Colonics

Person No.10
Has anyone done a colonic or are we cleansing our colons well enough? I hate the thought of those things but really want to be "cleaned out!"

Also, does this cleanse clean the liver or should I do a liver cleanse next?

Thanks for any input you can offer.

Peter
I have done colonics before the first Master Cleanse and done an herbal cleanse after the first MC as well to see the difference. I have found the Master Cleanse is the best for me and have no need for colonics. Others I've talked to like colonics and have done them after the Master Cleanse.

I think it comes back to the waste accumulating in layers in the colon. There are many years of waste in most people's colons and that takes several Master Cleanses or several series of colonics.

Although Burroughs warns against colonics and says they only clean out the last few feet of the colon (good point), the choice to use them is a personal one. The one thing I know with great certainty is that people's bodies are different and respond differently to treatment.

With regard to needing other cleanses after this one, see the topic "Cleansing, Other Types" above.

Cramping

Person No. 67
For those who suffer from unexplainable cramping, here's something to try. After reading the website on the benefits of cayenne pepper, I tried something and it worked immediately. I took a little more than one-half teaspoon of cayenne, put it on the back of my tongue, and

took a drink of lemonade. The cramping stopped instantly! I also had to eliminate immediately afterwards. It was like a miracle. It also worked with menstruation cramps.

Cravings

Person No. 30
I'm on the fifth day of my first MC. I've had this craving for milk — a cold, tall glass of milk — for the last three days. I've always been a milk drinker, but lately, I wasn't drinking as much. But now, I'm really craving it. Is this normal? It doesn't help because my son is a huge milk drinker too and our fridge is stocked with two whole gallons of milk! I wonder if I'll last another five days.

Person No. 21
Hi Person No.30: I'm on my fifth day too. I've craved Thai food since the beginning of the fast. I think the lemon along with the cayenne is reminding me of it. From what I've read cravings are pretty normal with this fast. You're half way there! Don't give in now. You can do it.

Person No. 1
It has been said that when you are having cravings your body is removing those toxins from your body and that the cravings will go away after your morning BMs.

This is Day 8 for me. I feel really great. Whatever mild cravings I had were gone by the evening hours of Day 5. Whatever you do, do not quit! You have completed the hardest part of the fast. Good luck!

Person No. 30
Thanks for the responses! You were right, my cravings have subsided.

Person No. 11
Hi everyone! Today is Day 3 for me on my first MC. I tried to start Monday but by dinnertime I gave in and ate! So, I started over. The first two days were really tough with the cravings. So, I had a cup of organic veggie broth each day! I wonder how badly that will impact my detoxing. I almost quit last night because we had family over for dinner and the smell of the food drove me insane! Today I woke up feeling okay. Anyway, I am glad I found this forum. Knowing that other people feel my "pain" will help me get through this. Good luck, everyone!

Peter

The first two days are the worst and trying to do it for the first time with family over and them cooking is heroic! Unfortunately, drinking veggie broth will only prolong the cravings and detox symptoms. Whatever the body is detoxing and eliminating is what you're craving. If you keep putting stuff in, it will continuously be eliminated and thus keep the cravings going. You want to avoid that.

Person No. 11

Thanks for the info, Peter. I will resist the temptation to drink the veggie broth! It's tough to do this, especially when my husband is crunching into an oooh-soo-delicious-sounding grilled cheese sandwich! Ah, this is so hard! Thank goodness I found this forum!

Daily Experiences

Person No. 1

This is Day 8 for me. I feel really good. No food cravings. Lots of energy. My tongue is clearing and my breath/mouth feels/smells good. My skin looks really good. The white portion of my eyes looks whiter than usual. If I feel okay at Day 10, I may extend my fast to fourteen days, but I'll take it one day at a time. I have not felt this great in years. I have passed *The Master Cleanser* book to a number of friends.

Person No. 11

I am on Day 4. I didn't wake up with huge cravings—and seeing a cup of coffee and a jar of peanut butter didn't drive me to seizures either! I feel a little icky, I woke up and my body just sort of ached. Interesting to note: last summer I got ringworm on my leg from a puppy my brother adopted from the Humane Society. I cured my leg by using essential oils and it went away, except I had a dark patch on my skin where I had it. On Day 2 of my cleanse, I was out shoveling snow (we got hit hard in Toronto this week). I thought I got frostbite because my leg was feeling just like I had burned it on the ringworm area. This lasted about two days. Today I woke up, no pain, and more importantly, no more dark patch of skin! Could this be part of the whole detox thing? I am feeling so happy! It's hard to explain: aside from the physical symptoms, this is turning out to be a very spiritual thing. I hope to be able to keep the positive attitude and make my goal of ten days! I hope you are all achieving great milestones as well! Hang in there and don't give up!

Person No. 11

I forgot to add that I stepped on the scale this morning and weighed five pounds less!!!

Person No. 10

Day 9, tongue is almost pink (actually was yesterday), short term memory sucks! Today I feel tired, possibly because it is Saturday so I am allowing it. Generally feel great, can move all joints freely and that is awesome!

I have lost thirteen pounds, but have done this many times before and do not do this for weight loss. I do it to cleanse and to return to good eating habits. However, I do want to lose at least seven more pounds.

Person No. 21

This is my first MC. I'm on Day 7 and feeling great. My tongue is already turning pink. It isn't perfectly pink but it is definitely clearing. I've been very generous with the cayenne in my lemonade. I wonder if that is helping to move things along. I love the taste of it. My sense of smell has greatly increased. My hubby and I took our boys to the Air and Space Museum yesterday and everywhere I turned I smelled halitosis.

I keep reading online about liver and parasite cleanses and wonder if I need that or not.

Peter

Burroughs says the Master Cleanse will cleanse all the organs and glands including the kidneys and liver. From experience, I know that the Master Cleanse handles parasites. Other nutritional, natural healers, including Norman Walker, have said parasites require waste accumulations in order to find good breeding grounds. So it makes sense that the Master Cleanse also handles parasites.

Person No. 8

Unfortunately, I had to get off of the cleanse on Day 6. I was just too hungry and getting hungrier all of the time, no matter how much lemonade or water I had. The first four days were fine and then I started getting hungry—very hungry. My husband just finished Day 10 and feels good. He had to stop the tea and the salt water for a couple of days because of work, but even though he did, he eliminated today. He said it was real black and really stunk. Good sign. He is getting rid of a lot of old toxins. He is shooting to go to twenty days. I don't really get cravings for SAD (Standard American Diet) foods but he does. We are hoping the cleanse will take care of those cravings.

Person No. 6

I am on Day 1. I chose to quit smoking and do the cleanse at the same time and I have never experienced a more pleasant experience quitting smoking. I hardly think of smoking at all because I've had these weird food cravings since last night in spurts. I'd crave certain foods so bad, I could smell them. Give me a choice between a cigarette and a Whopper and the Whopper wins! At any rate, it's just after 1:30 p.m. I've just polished off my third glass of lemonade. And I've had five BMs today, which left me really tired and lethargic for about an hour. And now I'm fine and, surprisingly, not hungry. I want to satiate some weird taste bud war going on in my mouth. Other than the few cramps I had this morning, my stomach is fine.

Person No. 31

I am on Day 4. This is my second attempt at MC. I stopped the first time at Day 3 because of my food cravings. For the past year, I have disciplined myself to stay away from certain foods so that makes this MC much easier. Instead of wanting a burger, I really just want a big salad. My stomach starts to cramp when I need to eliminate some toxins and then I go to the bathroom and they go away. I'm not really hungry at all and I have sufficient energy for the day's activities.

Person No. 11

I am experiencing the whole heightened sense of smell, too. I had a friend come over and he smelled like snot! He has good hygiene and I was baffled by this new thing. I couldn't bear to be too close to him because I could just smell this "congestion" smell emanating from him. I went to the mall and it was like hitting a brick wall. It smelled AWFUL!

● Person No. 6

I'm on Day 2 of the cleanse. I was doing soooo well today up until an hour ago when I had to help my little one prepare a tasty sandwich for herself. I did offer up a few new rules in my household, which may benefit others living with children.

Rule #1—No eating in the car!

Rule #2—No eating around mommy for first few days of the cleanse!

Rule #3—Mommy will not be cooking during the cleanse. (To supplement this rule, we went grocery shopping and stockpiled on favorite microwavable dinners, fresh fruits, veggies and goodies to make tasty sandwiches.) Mom's taking a break from cooking for a while.

In the long run, it's beneficial all around, because in my household we were never healthy eaters and this cleanse gives me the time to reflect on how to slowly but surely change bad eating habits to good eating habits.

Person No. 24

Hi folks. Day 3 for me. I feel much better than I did. Lots of muscle aches and lower back pain today. The first day I was really sick like the flu, with nightmares and anxiety the first night. Then my vertebrae started adjusting—just like early pregnancy! It's like everything is loose again. I felt much better yesterday, more bored than sick (also detox symptoms I hear) and today my body aches are the rule of the morning. I can't wait to see what freedom comes after these aches pass! I am really committed to ten days minimum. This fast has been too long in coming. I tried the MC four years ago and only made it a couple days and I have had adult acne ever since. My skin is already clearing up by Day 3. Think of all the time, grief and money I could have saved by just cleansing and changing my diet!! Have a great day!

Person No. 8

My husband is just finishing up Day 14. He is not hungry, just missing being able to chew food. Energy level normal. Since we eat 90% raw, he already is in pretty good shape. He has lost fifteen pounds so far. His tongue is just starting to look a little better. Not so coated. His breath is starting to smell not quite so bad. Boy, was that awful for awhile. He's shooting to go twenty days or less if his tongue turns pink first. Even though I didn't make it all ten days (only six since I kept getting hungrier and hungrier) I find that I am eating less and sleeping less with the same amount of energy I had before. So, all of you people just starting, hang in there. You won't regret it.

Person No. 6

Hi all, I'm on Day 5. What an accomplishment! I read somewhere that when you begin a fast your body is busy storing fat and water as it goes into save and protect mode. Then, anywhere from Day 3 to Day

71

5, your body actually begins the cleansing process and you will not feel hungry at this point. So, if this is Day 1 or 2 for you, please don't give up. It only gets easier! Good luck, all!

Person No. 12

Hi. I started Saturday morning, so today is my third day. The hardest part for me was Day 1 and 2. One word of advice, don't announce the cleanse to every person you meet to feed any ego that you may have or excitement to tell all. Don't argue with the uneducated. Don't try to convince other people until you educate yourself. Don't set yourself up for failure or negative feedback. I have only let a few close friends in on my great adventure. So far, so good! Best of luck to all and to all a spicy lemonade! Talk atcha soon.

Person No. 11

I actually prepared dinner tonight for my husband and daughter. While I acknowledge the fact that it would be nice to taste what I made, I was able to NOT TAKE A SINGLE NIBBLE! How's that for self-restraint?

Person No. 3

I am on Day 7. I can't believe I have made it this far. I will say that today is the first day I have had cravings of any kind. I am really hungry today and I had a lot of abdominal cramping. I am still debating whether to go twenty days. A part of me says go for it and a part of me says I miss food, especially when you go out to dinner with friends and family and you are the only one not eating. That happened four times this weekend!

Person No. 32

Today is Day 8 for me. So far today has been the best day. I feel serene, at peace. My thinking is shifting. It's really wonderful. I'm still a little tired in the evening, but I suppose that is to be expected. Or, if Peter is right, maybe tomorrow I won't be tired anymore. Hope so!

Person No. 16

Today would have been my ninth day but I had to quit because I was getting a little restless, but up until today I have been very into the MC, very happy, a lot of energy. But I'm glad today to get some fruit.

Peter

"Restlessness" is just another detox symptom, but I'm glad you had a good cleanse. When you feel like it, do another Master Cleanse. They just get easier and better.

Person No. 33

Day 9: Day 10 will begin once I go to bed. I have a rash on my face. I have gone through moments of feeling great, mentally fresh and feelings of exuberance. I really would like to go to Day 20. My goal is to continue until my face has cleared up. For me the bumps on my face are a detox symptom. My skin has always been very clear.

Person No. 18

I'm on Day 8 and I feel fantastic. I'm quite proud of myself and have even recruited about five others to do the cleanse. I had to call and encourage my sister and her husband last night. It was their first day and although they said it was rough they both seemed determined. I had a larger than usual BM this morning after a day of heavy cayenne pepper in the lemonade. All in all, life is good.

Person No. 18

I'm on Day 9 and I plan to go past the ten-day mark and shoot for at least fourteen. I was utterly amazed this morning at how much stuff came out. I concluded that the tea and salt water had really broken up a lot of my old intestinal waste. I definitely shed some layers this morning. If I can make it thru Superbowl weekend (it's here in Houston where I live) and all the festivities, then I think that twenty days might really be possible for me. That would be awesome for my first cleanse.

Person No. 33

I am on Day 13. My husband stopped on Day 11. I was feeling great. But, last night I began to have mucus. It surprised me somewhat because I thought the cleansing was done. I also have this annoying rash on my face. I thought that it was getting better but it seems to be moving about my face. If anyone has any idea what it may be from let me know. I thought maybe it was toxins, but now I don't know. I am committed to stay on the lemonade drink until the rash is gone. My plan is to stay until Day 20.

Peter

The body treats any cooked food and all meats, dairy, artificial colors, flavors and preservatives, alcohol, non-herbal tea, soda, beer, wine, tobacco and drugs as though they are poisons. It attempts to handle this condition by sending white blood cells (leukocytes). It also creates a layer of mucus in the colon to protect the body from absorbing these poisons directly into the blood stream.

As you release toxins on the cleanse, it is quite probable that the body is creating mucus to attempt handle the newly released toxins before they are eliminated. The handling, of course, would be to continue the cleanse or do another when time permits to eliminate more of the toxins.

The rash is also probably a result of the detox. That it is moving around on your face shows that change is happening. Detoxing is a change. We want that.

A friend had a history of hemorrhoids. On the second day of the cleanse (just three weeks ago) he got bleeding hemorrhoids, but they were not as painful as before. A few days later they went away. He feels they will never come back as long as he keeps his diet relatively clean.

Day 1

Person No. 13

First day on the cleanse. I have done a couple of fasts before, but not really anything close to this. The first fast I did only lasted a couple of days. I was drinking fresh veggie and fruit juice, but I became violently ill on the third day—vomiting and diarrhea. I don't believe this was due to the detox because I have been a raw vegan—with some cheating—for about seven months and I went through a bad detox period when I started as a vegan. I think what happened was that I let my veggie juice sit too long.

The second fast I did was six days, but it wasn't really complete because I ended up using some processed juices due to work/laziness. This did me some good but I have a feeling this fast will be much better.

I had initially planned to do this Master Cleanse for fourteen days, but I keep reading here that twenty days is optimal. So, I will try to make it for the twenty.

I have not done a salt flush yet. I am using the laxative tea so far, but I think I will try a salt flush tomorrow. I have yet to eliminate and don't know how much waste to expect, especially since I have been a raw foodist and things normally move through me very quickly. The last fast I did, I was still eliminating five days into it. That's a ton of backup. Now I tend to think I don't have a lot of backup, but then again I was on the SAD (Standard American Diet) for 22 years. There is no telling what's in there.

If there are any other short-term raw foodists here who have done this cleanse, I'd be curious to know how it affected you in general and how much waste you expelled/how quickly. Otherwise, I hope to stay positive and have no major problems doing this. I will post sometimes to update on my progress.

Person No. 27
This is my first day on the fast too, so I thought I would offer you support since I will need it myself! We are polar opposites as far as our normal diets. I have never even been a vegetarian, much less raw vegan. I am curious as to what sort of different results this fast will have on each of us. I was afraid I would be terribly hungry, but I have not been too hungry. Good luck!

Person No. 13
Thanks. Good luck to you too. My fast is either going really well or really bad depending on how I look at it. I'm in a lot of pain from burning BMs.

Peter
My first twenty-day Master Cleanse was after six months of a 100% raw vegetable/fruit/nut/seed diet. I had already lost over forty pounds on that diet and proceeded to lose another twenty on the Master Cleanse. I had burning BMs for four or five days and was amazed at all I had to get out.

I read your post, Person No.13, and given the reaction you are having now with the burning pain, I'd say you probably started a serious detox on your juice cleanse rather than a reaction from letting the veggie juice "sit too long."

I'm always quite surprised by who ends up having severe detox symptoms on the cleanse. Sometimes it's medications they took and/ or food they ate long before their current diet that caused the symptoms.

The solution is to emphasize the elimination part of the Master Cleanse. Drink lots of lemonade and the laxative tea, do the salt water flush and continue. If it gets really bad, discontinue the cleanse and eat raw fruits and vegetables to detox more slowly. You can always do the cleanse again later.

Person No. 13
Yes, my former habits explain a lot about the pain. Thanks.

Day 3—Feeling Good

● Person No. 14
Just wanted to say that I have reached Day 3 and am feeling surprisingly good. Day 1 and 2 were quite hard. Although I don't like to quit anything, last night I was tempted to cut this thing short. Today I feel very excited, enthusiastic and optimistic about everything. So my advice to anyone on Day 1 or 2 is just to get through it. It seems much better after those two hard days. The SWF (salt water flush) is awful, but I would say it is really important to do it. The results are fantastic. Good luck to everyone who is cleansing. It's a really good thing to do.

Person No. 12
Good for you. I agree. Day 1-3 were the worst for me. I started on a Saturday surrounded by kids and my hubby eating crap in front of me. Crap that I usually eat!! I am on Day 5 and this is my first MC. I have not had a solid movement yet, but I am looking forward to it. It's crazy but good that we can talk about our daily eliminations to each other.

This website helps me with support no one else understands! I can say though, my hubby has been supportive and proud of me. Good luck to you. Have you done this before? My goal is fourteen days. Ending my MC on January 30th unless I feel detoxified before that. Heck, I may keep going if need be!

Person No. 14
Thanks for all your lovely words of encouragement. This is my first MC. I became a raw foodist last August and that has been great. Christmas broke my willpower and I ate so much crap it was unreal. I took a look at myself a couple of weeks ago and I looked bad. My skin had broken out. I had cold sores and I felt terrible. So, I thought I

needed a good cleanout which is why I am doing this. Hopefully, it will put me on the straight and narrow again and I can go back to eating all my lovely raw food again. It's been hard for me cooking and watching my husband and two kids eat food. I think the masochist in me is making me cook all the foods that I really love. Fortunately, I have iron willpower and I won't give up. I am going to keep going for the ten days then I will see how I feel and maybe go a bit longer. It seems a shame to get so far and then stop when you know you need to detox a bit more. So who knows, I'll see how I feel next week. Lovely to talk to you and thanks for all your kind words.

Person No. 13
This is my third day too and while I am having some burning still, I feel ten times better than I did the past two days. In addition to pain, I also had so many toxins floating about that I was completely disoriented and couldn't concentrate on anything. I also slept a whole lot, but this is probably a good thing. I'm going to continue to twenty days. This is perfect because I will be ending on Saturday, Feb. 7th, then I can do fruit juice and some oranges on Sunday, and have my first big salad again on that Monday. Oh, how I look forward to that salad.

It's amazing how fast you start to see your face change after you cheat on your raw diet, isn't it? You get all puffy and pale, and lose the glow. The good thing is that you get it right back when you go back to 100% raw. I cheated for about a month straight on my raw diet, and boy did I look and feel bad.

I can't say I am perfect. I cheat every now and then, but the rewards never add up. It only makes me feel bad and remember why I went raw to begin with. Good luck!

Person No. 14
You are so right about the face. I've just been to the bathroom and as I turned round—I have a big mirror—I have just this minute thought to myself how much better my face is looking–not quite so old somehow. How long have you been raw? At times I find it quite a challenge. Especially if I'm facing some stress—that old thing of reaching for food when you're under stress. Overall though I love how it makes me look and feel and it makes so much sense. It's nice to talk to someone else who has found raw food. I am the only person where I live who is into it. I think most people think I'm a little extreme.

So, it's great to find a like-minded person. I think we may have strayed from the topic of the Master Cleanse, but I guess it's sort of related. Good luck on Day 4 and on reaching your goals.

● Peter

Clear skin is an indicator that you are no longer overloading your digestive system with toxins that have to be eliminated. One of the major organs of elimination, and the largest, is the skin. When you cease putting cooked food, meat, dairy, artificial colors, flavors and preservatives into your body, your skin clears up quickly as it no longer needs to eliminate "junk," which is what makes your skin look old and ill.

Person No. 13

I have been raw for almost eight months—really seven because I cheated almost every day for one entire month. I do cheat occasionally, and yes it is normally in times of stress, going back to old comforts, etc. Sometimes I allow myself to cheat because I feel I deserve it, which is silly because I'm saying that I deserve to mess my body up. I also know that I recover fast and when I do cheat, I don't cheat badly. I usually only eat cooked veggies. Bread and rice make me horribly ill.

Yes, it is looked upon as extreme and I am the only person here as well who is raw or even vegan. However I have a couple of friends online who give me support and that helps. Otherwise, I just know that this is the best thing to do—the only thing that makes sense and gives you proper nourishment. It's simple. It's called nature, but most people are so conditioned from birth that this natural way of eating seems totally preposterous to them. I guess we are getting on a different topic.

I try my best and generally feel great. I know I'll feel even better after I do this cleanse. I'm so glad this bulletin board is here. It helps a lot to keep me going because this thing is no picnic, but I know it will be worth it in the end.

Peter

It's always nice to run into more people who are eating a raw veggies/fruits/nuts/seeds diet. My wife and I do also. Here in Clearwater, Florida, we have a raw food group with health food stores, a support group, and occasional monthly potluck dinners.

One benefit I gained from my twenty-day cleanse was the ability to face stress without handling it with food. I recommend the longer cleanse for clearing a person's mind and putting your life goals in perspective.

Day 5

Person No. 1

This is Day 5 for me. As I mentioned previously, I had a sore throat for the past day and a half and itchy inner ears. Well, IT'S ALL GONE AWAY! I just have a runny nose (clear mucus)—no thick stuff yet. I guess I was pretty toxic after all. This is my first time doing the MC. I am convinced that the MC is the right thing to do for overall good body health. I will do this the recommended three to four times a year for life. I will also modify my diet. I have asthma so I have concerns as to what detox symptoms I will experience as a result of it while on the MC.

Person No. 10

Day 5 for me too and I feel great. I have done this so many times and have never felt as good as when I am on the cleanse. It was as if my body had seized up and is now releasing and I can move freely again. I am going to continue until my tongue is pink (although this time it isn't as bad as other times when it got a thick yellow coating).

I am not doing the salt water flush as the last couple of times I gagged but instead am drinking laxative tea night and morning and I am definitely "flushing."

Person No. 34

Today is Day 7 for me. The first four days were very good—I felt good. Then on Day 5 I started to feel really horrible with stomachaches and stuff. I continued the cleanse and on Day 6 the symptoms started to go away. Now, I'm feeling a lot better. The good things I've noticed so far are my face is clearing up, I feel much more energized, my plugged left ear cleared up and my sinus infection went away! I was planning to go the ten days but I might go a little longer to fully clear up my tongue. It was the most white yesterday but today it's less. So, we'll see.

Day 10!

Person No. 21

I'm on my tenth day of the MC and I think I'm going to keep on going. It is kind of funny, when I started I was determined to make ten days, but felt it would be really hard. I was even planning what kind of food I would treat myself to when I was done (Thai Food). Now, I really feel the need to get rid of more toxins. I woke up this morning with a lot of nasal mucus. I think this is going to be a big detox day and I really don't think I should end the fast that way. I want to be completely clear. I've had so many improvements in my health along the way. I have no need for my asthma or allergy meds. My eczema is clearing and I have no acne. I'm no longer eating when I'm confronted with stressful situations. So onward I must go. Thanks for all of your help everyone.

Peter

Wow, Person No. 21, you're inspiring! I can identify with all that. I won't quit on a detox day and I like Thai food when I'm not eating raw.

Person No. 11

Hi everyone! It is now Day 10 for me and I am sooo excited! I can't believe I made it through. My tongue is not completely pink yet. I had thought about extending the fast, but since it is my first time, I will be a wimp and finish it today. Yes, I do miss food a lot! I am really looking forward to that veggie salad or soup. I lost a total of nine pounds. I was a little disappointed that it wasn't more but realistically, I am 5'1" and down to 106 pounds. So, any more probably wouldn't be healthy. I would love to hit the 99-100 pound mark though. Ah, the college days! Maybe if I extend the fast I would lose more, but I want to keep the reason for the fast in perspective and it was never to lose weight to begin with. I would like to know from people who have done this before, did they gain all the weight back? How long did it take? I am curious and a little scared. I am attached to my rib count now! Anyway, thanks for all the support everyone, best of luck on the MC and I will probably be back in a few months to do it all over again!

Person No. 6

You go girl! Victory!

Peter

You raise a good question about regaining the weight. I lost a little more than twenty pounds on my first twenty-day cleanse. I then stayed on mostly raw veggies/fruit/nuts/seeds with occasional forays into ribs, ice cream and the bad stuff for fun. I'd say I was about 90–95% raw. I then did two more ten-day cleanses just because I liked them. By then it was a year later and my weight was about the same as when I finished the first cleanse. Before the first cleanse, I ate a 100% raw veggie, etc. diet for six months and lost 46 pounds! None of that has come back. Before I went raw veggie, etc. I couldn't quite get into my 40-inch waist pants. Now I fit easily into 34s.

It's all about what you eat. If you eat the "bad stuff," which the body sees as toxins, the body will protect itself by making mucus to line the digestive tract and store the toxins in the body fat. That's just how it is. Eat junk and get fat. If you eat real food, food with nutritive value, you will lose to an ideal weight and not gain it back at all. There you go: total control of your weight and health.

Person No. 12

I just wanted to say thanks to everyone (especially Peter) for all the advice and support. I have entered into Day 10 and I am going for Day 14! I figure I'm already here and I have no more weekends to get through. I might as well.

I have seen great results. For everyone out there doubting it or wanting to quit, hold out! Not only is it a great test of will, it is overall the best feeling of good health you'll ever experience! Your sense of food appreciation grows tremendously and self discipline is at its highest. Respect for your body (temple) is found quickly. We are what we eat—how true, how true. Thanks again. God bless.

Person No. 10

Thank you to everyone for your words of encouragement, knowledge and shared experiences. I am now on Day 11 and I feel terrific! I am quitting today but staying on broth for ten days. I would like to lose a few more pounds and really get committed to my health. I don't trust that if I return to normal eating today I will "behave," so the broth option is great for me.

My skin is so clear and glowing. I've lost fifteen pounds. I am at peace and proud of myself! I have done this at least ten times before and this was the easiest ever. Good health and happiness to you all for 2004 and beyond.

Day 10, Beyond

Person No. 10
I am on Day 8 and feel great. My joints are all moving freely and my arthritic pains are just about gone. I was prepared to stay on the cleanse for as long as it took for my tongue to turn pink, but it is pink already. So, I will probably just stay for the ten days unless there is a further benefit I don't know about. Thanks for all your assistance, Peter.

● Peter
I would divide the benefits of going beyond the tenth day into two categories. The first are spiritual in nature. I found a sense of serenity, an increased ability to confront and handle problems, and the absence of desire to eat "bad" food even while I could appreciate and enjoy the smell of it. The idea of consuming something that would be bad for my body even though it smelled good was like the idea of eating a scratch n' sniff sticker. You would not even think of it.*

The second category of gain depends on whether there's more waste to be eliminated. That would be personal. I will tell you that the three other people I personally know who have done more than ten days in a row on the cleanse, say they had their biggest benefits from the additional days.

*For the record, I occasionally eat unhealthy things just for the fun of it. However, the vast majority (more than 90%) of food I eat is fresh, raw real food with nutritional value and no added preservatives, additives, colors, poisons, etc. I have also leaned that when I do eat "bad" food I can just do the salt water flush the next day, if I feel bad. I also know I can hit the body's "reset button" by doing a Master Cleanse, which for me and others I know, gets the body back to wanting healthy food and juices.

● Detox Symptoms—Don't Hate Them: They Are Milestones

Peter

Although detoxification symptoms are unpleasant, they ought to be desired. No one wants the feelings associated with detoxifying, but that's the purpose of the cleanse. If you are not detoxifying, you are not making progress and will not feel better afterward!

I place detox symptoms into five classes. I went into these earlier in the book, and reiterate them here. Knowing these symptoms will be gone in a day or two, it is much easier to persevere and complete the cleanse.

1. **Cravings**. I've noticed I crave things for a few hours or a day. Usually after the next morning's elimination, the craving is gone and I feel better. As your body detoxifies (eliminates the toxic waste from) cooked meat, dairy products, etc., it craves the hamburger, pizza, ice cream, etc. that is being "peeled off" in layers.

2. **Tiredness**. When your body fights toxins, whether from detoxifying or an infection, it diverts energy into healing and away from the energy you use to work and play. Sleep is a natural refuge at these times. This happens only occasionally on the Master Cleanse, but can occur chronically in those who eat diets that are mostly toxic, that contain artificial colors, flavors, preservatives, additives, pesticides, fertilizers, or environmental contamination not washed off the food before eating.

3. **Irritability, boredom, etc.** This includes the desire to "just chew something solid."

4. **Physical aches, pains, nausea, vomiting, etc.** These are the most severe reactions and only occur where a person is severely toxic; only a small percentage of people (perhaps 1%) experience these. Fortunately, these have gone away after only a day or two in every case I have heard about.

5. **Hot or burning bowel movements**. Toxins and other waste are acidic. I have found that when I eliminate old waste and other toxins, my bowel movements are actually hot. During my first Master Cleanse, my eliminations actually burned. I have also

noticed that when I have serious detox symptoms as listed above, my eliminations the next morning are typically hot.

Now that you know these are only temporary and are milestones that you are becoming healthier, you will have the perspective to complete the cleanse and make it through. After you personally experience the gain you make after a detox day, you'll actually begin to look forward to them, knowing that the next day will be a new plateau!

Diabetics, Special Instructions

Peter
I've had a number of people with diabetes ask about doing the Master Cleanse. Burroughs instructs diabetics to use only a tablespoon of molasses in the lemonade at first and gradually increase the amount until they are using two tablespoons. He also recommends regular checks of the sugar level in the urine and blood to monitor insulin requirements as they change. Upon completing the Master Cleanse, a diet of fresh raw vegetables, nuts, seeds and fruits is recommended.

Not being a doctor myself, you should discuss these instructions with your health professional.

Diarrhea

Person No. 35
I'm starting my second day of the MC. Yesterday went fine and I drank the tea before bed. I had a restless night of sleep as my tummy was "rumbly" all night. I could only get down one-half the salt water this morning, so I am making more laxative tea. I already have diarrhea. Is this normal? Should I drink more tea?

Peter
Is this actually diarrhea or just four or five watery bowel movements from the salt water? If it's really diarrhea, discontinue the salt water and/or any morning laxative tea until the diarrhea is gone.

Person No. 35
Unfortunately it's the real deal along with incredible cramping. So, are you saying I should stop the laxative tea till the diarrhea subsides?

I haven't been able to find the book locally. I am going to order it today. In the meantime, I really appreciate the bulletin board to answer questions. Today is much more challenging than yesterday. But I just kept reminding myself that you said the symptoms will most likely subside with the next morning's flush. Thanks for the encouragement.

Peter
Yes, if you have the real deal, follow Burrough's advice and discontinue the laxative tea and salt water until the diarrhea is gone. The first couple of days are usually the worst, then around the seventh day. I am glad you are sticking with it.

Emotional Detox?

Person No. 35
Hi Everyone. It sure helps to read how everyone is doing. I am just about through Day 4 and, like many of you, I'm wondering if I'll make it. My hunger comes and goes, same with the cravings. I seem to be craving things I don't normally eat, which I find comical: pizza, bratwurst, a ham and cheese sandwich.

Day 2 was a physical detox day for me and today, Day 4, has felt like an emotional detox. Has anyone else experienced an "emotional detox?" I had a dream just before I woke up that triggered the various fears I've been carrying around for weeks. They all surfaced en masse today and I found I just had to face them and deal with them. I'm doing better this evening.

As far as elimination goes, the only thing I'm eliminating is bile. I'm on my third day of diarrhea and not doing the salt water or the laxative tea. Is anyone else having this issue? Thanks for this site, everyone.

Peter
I've had plenty of "emotional detox days" and so have others. (See the topic "Detox Symptoms—Don't Hate Them: They Are Milestones.")

What I found on the twenty-day cleanse was that the second ten days was learning to handle problems without turning to food. In addition to that valuable lesson, I also gained a much more pleasant and even-tempered disposition. I think that these benefits are perhaps the reasons many religions and Indian tribes use fasts to help the spiritual nature of man.

Regarding the diarrhea, your body is getting rid of wastes. As long as it doesn't continue for more than four or five days, I'd continue. If it goes on beyond that, you should probably discontinue the cleanse. If that doesn't stop it, you should see a health professional. Diarrhea can be serious if it continues for a long time.

Person No. 12
Some may call it an emotional detox. I call it a spiritual breakthrough.

Headaches on the Cleanse

Peter
Having talked to perhaps six or eight people who experienced headaches on the first few days of the cleanse, I want to pass on what I've learned.

Coming off a heavy caffeine (coffee, sodas, or tea) habit on the cleanse frequently causes headaches even in people who eat healthy food and are otherwise in good shape. If you are coming off coffee, be sure to have six to twelve drinks of the lemonade each day along with plenty of water to wash out the toxins. In addition, be sure to follow the instructions on the salt water flush and the laxative tea. You want to eliminate as many of the toxins as fast as you can.

Most important of all, recognize that the headaches are detox symptoms from quitting coffee (or other caffeine addictions). They usually go away within four days.

Person No. 34
I used to drink one to two cups of coffee daily before I did the cleanse the first time. The first day of the cleanse that time, I had the worst headache I think I've ever had. By the second day it was just barely there and by the third it was completely gone. I never returned to a daily ritual of a morning coffee since the first cleanse, so when I started the cleanse the second time I had no headache at all this time.

Person No. 2

I can relate to the headache. I've concluded it was my coffee addiction. I did a MC in May and didn't have the headaches that I did this time, but I started drinking coffee in September and was having two or more cups a day with about four or more cups of Earl Grey tea. I definitely feel it was coffee. I craved coffee the first three days. Woke up Day 4, no craving and no headache.

Check your tongue. You'll see how white it is to go with the headache. Hang in there—my headache went away totally by Day 4. Make sure you are getting lots of lemonade and water. My error was drinking only four lemonades. Still can't get beyond that, but made up with water.

Person No. 36

This will be the first MC fast for my spouse and me. She had a question regarding headaches. She has to take something every day for headaches, usually Sudafed, or the headache will go into a migraine. She is concerned that when we start the fast the headaches will become unbearable. What should she do?

Peter

First, she must get off any caffeine products: soft drinks, coffee, etc. They always produce headaches as the person comes off the addiction. Then when she does the cleanse, she must keep in all the elimination steps: herbal laxative tea, salt water flush, lots of lemonade (six to twelve ten-ounce drinks a day) and plenty of water. If the headaches get to be too much, she can always go off the cleanse and take whatever she needs.

Honey vs. Maple Syrup

Person No. 69

Can honey be substituted for maple syrup?

Peter

Burroughs says never use honey internally. It is predigested by bees and goes directly into the blood stream—like alcohol—spiking blood sugar and prompting the body to reduce it by secreting insulin, which lowers the blood sugar, which promotes depression.

I wouldn't go as far as to say never to use honey internally. However, I don't use or recommend people substituting honey for maple syrup for the Master Cleanse.

Person No. 69
What is the purpose of the maple syrup? Is it for energy?

Peter
Yes, plus the maple syrup provides many minerals, including sodium, potassium, calcium, magnesium, and others. It also provides Vitamins A, B_1, B_2, B_6, C and Pantothenic Acid (B_5).

Hungry

Person No. 14
I am now on Day 7. To be honest the first three days were the best in terms of not being hungry. It has steadily gotten worse. Yesterday and today I am starving. Is this another detox sign? I thought hunger subsided. I am not craving anything. It's just a gnawing hunger and my stomach is constantly rumbling—even after the lemonade. Anyone else like this?

Person No. 70
I was in the same boat. The first time I did the cleanse I only lasted until Day 9 and was so hungry I couldn't stand it. I did everything the way I should have too. This time I tried to add more water. Drink a lemonade, drink a water. By Day 6, I was just getting hungrier and more miserable. So, I quit. Wish I could do it to Day 10, but for some reason I can't handle it. I had the same problem when I did a juice fast.

Peter
Hunger as you describe it sounds to me like you are not getting enough lemonade or water. I have read that a single glass of water will turn off hunger in more than 90% of people on diets. Since you can have six to twelve glasses of the lemonade per day and as much water as you want, you should be able to fill your stomach easily.

After this bulletin board exchange, while writing this book, I learned something else about people experiencing hunger. I was able to reach two people who experienced hunger, not cravings, and both had taken diet pills for some years. Therefore I think in some cases, the hunger was due to detoxification of the residue from the diet pills.

So I now know of four possibilities for hunger: 1) The person is not drinking another glass of lemonade or water, 2) The person is eating or drinking something other than the lemonade, salt water, or tea and that is creating his/her cravings the next day; 3) The person is perceiving cravings as hunger; or 4) The person has a history of diet pills.

Interrupting the Cleanse

Peter
People have asked if they could "break" the cleanse with orange juice and/or grapefruit juice for a few days and then get back on it without losing the weight loss and cleansing benefits. I do not recommend it. Just orange juice or grapefruit juice might be okay for one day, but it will not sustain you for many days in a row.

January Cleanse

[In the middle of December 2003, my wife and I decided to promote a Master Cleanse in January 2004 to help people recover from the excesses of the holidays. I had set a goal of 100 people doing the cleanse that month. We actually had 110 people on the bulletin board cleansing and I knew of ten more that did not have a connection to the Internet. So, they could not post to the bulletin board.]

Person No. 10
I've done this many times and love it. My experience has always been about the same—one or two days of discomfort, headaches and hunger. The next few days are great and then Days 8 onward are fantastic. It is more than about food. It becomes about how blessed I am in all areas of my life. God Bless and Happy New Year!

Person No. 37
I am so happy to see several people with the same idea as I have. I am starting the Master Cleanse today and plan on doing it quarterly. It's the best thing for my body. I felt great after my first cleanse.

Person No. 38

I am going to start my first time Master Cleanse on Monday, the 5th of January. My husband says he's going to do it with me. I hope so since he's seen what a difference a recent raw food/juice cleanse did for me at an institute in San Diego, where a raw foods lifestyle was introduced to me. I love the way it made me feel and want to incorporate more of it into our lives. I was happy to find your website. Thank you.

Person No. 39

I am on Day 9. One more day left, then orange juice and soup! I've had these wonderful things happen to me while on the cleanse:

1.   I lost 10 lbs.

2.   I no longer have to get surgery on knee as the toxin buildup is gone!

3.   My blemishes cleared up and my overall skin is soft and smooth.

4.   I had a mental, physical, and spiritual awakening!

This worked GREAT for me! I'm looking forward to organic food!

Person No. 40

I'm on my fourth day, I feel great and have really begun to notice a change in my sensory conditions, i.e. smell, taste, hearing, etc. WOW!

Person No. 7

I'm on Day 6 and feel very relaxed and in touch with my surroundings. This is my second attempt to do the Master Cleanse. The first time I was doing shift work and found it too difficult to go through the whole ten days. After speaking to many friends and reading all your comments, I came to the conclusion this is something I must experience. Drinking the lemonade is great. I love lemons, maple syrup and spicy foods. My cravings have finally disappeared and I am anxious to see what changes my body will go through in the next few days. Good health to all.

Person No. 41

I just want to let you know that I will be starting the cleanse tomorrow—January 16. This bulletin board has already been a real encouragement to me in my quest for healthy eating. I would like to become a raw vegan this year and this fast seems like the best way to start. I've read quite a bit about fasting and this seems to put a lot of the concepts together in a very workable method, so I guess I'll find out. I'm working on my husband and others to try to get them to participate in this fast also. We'll see if I can bump the number up. I'll be checking back in. Thanks.

Person No. 24

I am having a hard time drinking enough lemonade. I only drank four cups yesterday and only two so far today and it's already 4:00 p.m. Any thoughts? I look forward to more communing with the Master Cleansers! Love and light.

Person No. 11

What I have done to make sure I drink at least six glasses is I have left four lemons on my kitchen counter (four small lemons are enough for six glasses of lemonade). If they are gone by the end of the day, I know I have done okay. Good luck. I am on Day 5 and feeling great!

Person No. 24

Thank you so much for responding! I was feeling at a loss when I looked up to see if anyone had responded to me. Support helps a lot! Great to hear Day 5 is good. I think I will go take a shower and maybe a walk. If I can just make it through tonight, I will deal with tomorrow when it comes.

Peter

The first two or three days are always the worst because the toxins from the most recent waste are right there to be eliminated and when the toxins are eliminated, the body craves whatever is in the toxins: hamburgers, cheese, etc. So, it's usually easy to do the rest of the cleanse.

Person No. 17

I decided to get in on the January cleanse. This has been my first-ever day on my first-ever cleanse. It went okay, except I am already bored of the lemonade. Oh well, one day at a time. Gonna drink my lax tea and hit the sack. Thanks for the bulletin board. It is very helpful.

Peter

Boredom is a detox symptom. When you get past the first two or three days, you'll feel wonderful. That's your natural state. Boredom is the result of toxins in your body.

Person No. 12

Count me in your January "100." I started January 17, 2004. A friend of mine introduced it to me and she's a couple days ahead of me. We are a support system. My husband won't do it, but he is being very supportive. I love this site and I will continue to post questions and comments. I am on Day 3, slightly hungry, but in complete control so far. Reading the board, I see it gets better with time. Thank goodness!

Person No. 32

Hi Peter,

I met you at the raw food meeting in Clearwater this month and was planning on a three-day water fast, but after hearing you speak, I decided to do the Master Cleanse with a friend who was also at the meeting. You can count us in as part of the 100. We are on Day 6.

Prior to starting the cleanse, I ate just fruits and vegetables for three days in an attempt to cleanse a bit so that I wouldn't have bad toxic symptoms from all that sugar I ate at during the holidays. I was feeling headachy the night before the cleanse, and the entire first day. It was pretty bad and I really laughed at myself when I contemplated taking aspirin. The next morning, the headache traveled to the other side of my head, but by mid-morning it was gone. What a relief!

My aunt visited for the first five days of my fast, and left this morning. It was hard feeding her and my children—not seeing the food, but smelling it. I find that it makes me irritable to smell the food and not eat it. I suppose that's common. I'm hanging in there. Thanks for being here!

Peter

A pure raw vegetable and fruit diet also detoxifies. If you don't handle the other side of the program (elimination), you can end up with detox symptoms like headaches, irritability, boredom, cravings, etc. It's actually easier just to do the cleanse.

As far as it being difficult to feed others, that usually disappears around Day 8. A good friend, after Day 7, helped a friend of his, a chef, prepare grilled pork tenderloins for dinner and my friend on the cleanse wasn't bothered at all!

Thanks for posting on this bulletin board. It helps others to know how many are doing this. For example, this board was started on 29

Dec 2003 and already (21 Jan 2004) over 1100 (not a typographic error) people have read this topic!

Person No. 42
I am on Day 3 of my cleanse. I just found this site, it has already answered some of the things I was wondering about.

Person No. 32
Today is Day 8 and I'm happy to report that making dinner for my kids tonight didn't bother me at all. I am also extremely pleased to say that there has been a shift in my thinking today—about lots of things. I am much more serene and peaceful. The spiritual side of the fast is emerging and it feels wonderful! Thanks again for this board.

Person No. 43
Hello, I just completed my first day of the cleanse and intend to go more than ten days if possible. I have this strange ambition to do a forty-day cleanse. Odd, huh?

Peter
It's not a strange thought at all. I've often wondered about doing a forty-day cleanse myself. The benefits after Day 8 for me have all been spiritual: more clarity of purpose; the ability to face stress without turning to food as a comfortable avoidance mechanism; the ability to smell wonderful smells (ribs for me) without the compulsion to eat it—much like you wouldn't eat a bar of soap or a scratch n' sniff just because it smelled good. Many native cultures use fasts as a spiritual tool.

Person No. 33
My husband and I have joined the January cleanse. We are on Day 9. It is the first time for us both. I have fasted many times but was unable to do the lemonade fast before because I felt sick each time I tried. I was happy to find your website to hear about your challenge and am happy to report this time has been a success.

It has been a great challenge. The first three days found us in the bathroom often. My husband is about to stop and will be undertaking a raw food diet. I have decided to stay a few more days. I have been monitoring my detox and I believe I have some more time to go. I have a slight headache this morning. A few days ago I had drainage from my eyes and there appears to be a rash on my face. So I think I will continue until the rash goes away and my face clears up. Thanks for the challenge.

Peter
Good for you!

A detox day (rash, drainage, etc.) is not a day to stop. You'll be happy afterward.

Person No. 44
I am on Day 6 and I feel great. I am amazed that I did this. I am a construction worker and a bathroom is not always available so I must end my cleanse before I go back to work in three days. Today I will have orange juice. I already made the vegetable soup for tomorrow. I wish I could stay on this cleanse for more days as I feel better each day. I can breathe better and the dry skin on my hands has disappeared. I am shocked at what still leaves my body as I have not had food for six days. Gross!

Peter
Many people are in the same situation. See the "Salt water flush" topic for a quote about using herbal laxative tea morning and evening rather than drinking the salt water. Then you could stay on the cleanse longer. The spiritual and mental clarity starts for me around Day 8.

Laxative Tea

Person No. 12
For Your Information: I am on Day 7. I was using a laxative tea that came in a cleanse pack that I purchased before this cleanse (parasite cleanse). I did not get nearly the great results I did when I switched to Smooth Move. It was about $3.49 at my nearest health food store. When I compared both teas Smooth Move had more senna in it than the other tea I was using. I suggest Smooth Move. To each his own — just make sure the tea has enough senna.

Person No. 3
This is my first time and I am on Day 2. I really haven't seen or felt any different, although I can barely get half of the salt water flush down. I have a question about the tea. Can I use any laxative tea or does it have to be a specific one? Thanks. This board has been very helpful.

Peter

No special one is recommended by Burroughs. I recommend a tea with about 50% senna leaf. You can find them at your local health food store.

Person No. 7

Cascara Sagrada is a beneficial herb (it's actually bark) that I have used and found it to be milder than senna. I took it in capsule form. I don't think it should effect the cleanse. Just take lots of water along with it.

Peter

Senna can be too powerful when there is not much in the colon to expel. Switch to a senna blend (50% senna and 50% other herbs) or make only half a cup of senna and then dilute it with mint tea or water. Cascara Sagrada is not a good solution as it is too bitter to make into a tea and taking it in capsules (the usual method) requires digestion and slows the cleanse.

Person No. 45

I'm planning to start the cleanse on Saturday, but I have a concern regarding the SWF and laxative tea: after doing the flush and taking the tea for as long as I do the cleanse, is there a danger that my bowel will have become dependent on these, leading to problems after the cleanse?

Peter

Although I've had two other people ask that same question, I've never known of anyone to whom that actually happened.

Laxative Tea and Abdominal Cramps

Peter

I originally recommended senna tea as the laxative tea for the cleanse. Since then, I've learned that senna tea is very strong and can cause cramps. I've even had some cramps myself occasionally, but never thought anything of it.

However, on rereading *The Master Cleanser*, I found that Burroughs never specifies "senna." He only says herbal laxative tea. Now I recommend an herbal laxative tea blend with senna being only 50% of the ingredients.

When I first began my cleanses, my large colon was sluggish and the muscular contraction that moved the food along (peristalsis) was very weak. Now my elimination is great. So, the senna tea worked fine. Now, however, I use a senna blend. The one I like the most is Smooth Move by Traditional Medicinals. Yogi Tea makes another good one called Get Regular.

If you only have senna, you might try making only half a cup and watering it down by half. On the other hand, if you're not eliminating much of anything, you might want to try pure senna tea for a few days.

Lemonade, Amount to Drink

Person No. 46
This is my second day. When I mix up a pitcher of the lemonade, can I just pour myself a glass whenever I want, as long as I drink up to twelve glasses a day? Thank you! It's only my second day, but I feel such a great change already.

Peter
Yes, you can drink the lemonade whenever you want except I would wait at least a half hour after the salt water and would finish drinking the lemonade a couple hours before going to sleep so you don't have to wake up to pee. Then drink the laxative tea just before you go to sleep. But these are my suggestions only.

Lemonade, Premixing

Person No. 47
Do any of you premix a jug of lemonade to take to work with you, or is this a definite no-no?

Person No. 8
I don't know if it is a no-no or not but I make up a gallon at a time. Then I put it all in eleven-ounce bottles I have so I can just grab a

couple of bottles and go out the door. Today I went shopping and took two bottles of juice and two of water and I was gone for six hours. I was hungry when I got home but just made and drank some more. Good luck.

Peter

Let's face it. You have to do enough to go through the day if you're going to go to work outside your house. However, I have heard of people squeezing lemons (never use commercial bottled juice! It's pasteurized and old) and mixing the maple syrup as a "premix" that they then add to water over the next two or more days. If you've read anything about the wheatgrass diet, the Hippocrates diet, the raw food diet, the Gerson anti-degenerative disease regimen, juicing for health or the Optimum Health Institute, you know that enzymes diminish over time, even in as little time as a few hours.

You can't get away from having to make enough to get through the day, but making more than one day's supply (even a day and an evening) will diminish your benefits.

Person No. 34

I like to have my juice really fresh to get the full benefit of the enzymes in the lemons. However, I work an eight-hour day. So, what I do is make up a batch for just work. I usually drink three to four servings in that time. I do the lemon, maple syrup and water but not the cayenne pepper yet. I then pour myself one serving in a portable cup and add the pepper to just the one glass. Otherwise, the pepper gets too hot. When I pour myself a new glass at work, I add the pepper to that glass. Then when I come home at the end of the day, I just make one serving at a time.

Lemons, Buying in Quantity

Person No. 9

I'm starting the cleanse this weekend and after reading the topics, it looks like it's going to take around six or seven lemons a day. What is the shelf-life of lemons for the purpose of the cleanse? (I'm not sure if the beneficial properties break down while they are in the fridge.)

Also, I don't see too many people mentioning limes. Is there a big difference? Can you alternate just to shake things up a bit? Thanks!

Peter

A large lemon will yield two ounces of juice. So, for eight drinks a day, you will need four large lemons per day or forty for ten days. Organic lemons are good for about five days in the refrigerator.

Limes are great for a change of pace. They're smaller and you'll need about twice as many of them to make a drink. Burroughs says you can use either lemons or limes. I prefer the taste of lemons for the long run, but occasional drinks with lime are kind of fun.

Lemons, Juicing

Person No. 43

I'm on Day 5 and eating just seems so trivial at this point. I feel great and my energy is off the charts. I found a way of satisfying that need for "something solid." When I make my lemonade, instead of squeezing the lemon, I just blend it in a blender (without the peel). The pulp gives me the sensation that I'm eating something whole. Come to think of it, is that okay? I figured it would be, seeing as how some people blend the pulp and peel into the drink.

Peter

Yes, blending some of the skin (organic lemons only) and pulp can enhance the work of the lemon.

Person No. 14

Maybe a stupid question. Does it make any difference to the effectiveness of the lemons how you squeeze them? I have been using a Champion juicer and getting quite a bit of juice that way, but last night I couldn't be bothered to do it that way and used a plain old lemon squeezer. The juice tasted different. Anyone know if there's a best way or if it makes no difference?

Peter

I've done it both ways: using an expensive juicer with whole organic lemons and with just squeezing the lemons. The taste is quite different, but I got the same results both ways.

Person No. 21

This bulletin board is a wonderful source for information and support. I've really enjoyed reading the posts. I have a question. Is it ok to use "bottled" lemon juice instead of fresh organic lemons? I've been using fresh lemons, but I'm going through them fast and where I live lemons are kind of expensive. Also, are there inexpensive places to buy the organic maple syrup and lemons?

Peter

Bottled juice is a no-no as the vitamins and enzymes that do the good work are destroyed by time, sunlight and cooking (pasteurizing).

Concerning the high prices of organic ingredients for the cleanse, my wife and I figured that it's about $7.50 per day including the cost of maple syrup, lemons, sea salt and laxative tea. Well worth it. When you finish the cleanse, you'll discover that you don't eat as much quantity any more, so rather than eat foods that have had all their enzymes and vitamins removed and then had preservatives and pesticides added, why not spend the same money for fewer high-quality (organic) foods with real nutrition? One of the things I've learned from my research into nutrition and healing is that proper nutrition equals a pleasant, serene attitude toward life. The spiritual side starts to show through.

Person No. 48

Peter, I read your article in *Natural Awakenings* magazine and am so excited to start the cleanse! Must you use organic lemons or limes or can you just not use the rinds? Thanks so much.

Peter

It is not required to use organic lemons or limes. If you're only squeezing them and not putting them through a juicer, you needn't peel the rind on non-organic ones. That is only if you are going to put the whole thing through the juicer.

Length of Fasts and Time between Them

Person No. 49

How often should one do the cleanse? Is there a difference between a five-day and a twenty-day fast?

Peter

Burroughs says to do it for a minimum of ten days and he recommends doing it three to four times a year. I am on my third full cleanse in less than two years. Not only does this cleanse make the body healthier, but it also gives a wonderful peace of mind and sense of peaceful energy. My first cleanse was for twenty days. I have also done this cleanse for two and three days. Burroughs is right about doing it for at least ten days. The real gains start after Day 7 (a major detox day for me) and a twenty-day cleanse produces spiritual gains beyond just health. This cleanse is like pressing reset for the body. It puts everything back to normal.

Person No. 50
Peter, what is a major detox day? What are your symptoms? Thanks

Peter
A major detox day is one where you have noticeable symptoms. [See the topic "Detox symptoms—don't hate them; they are milestones" for more info.]

Person No. 16
Is there anything unhealthy about doing the cleanse and eating raw food on alternate days? It would keep my body clean and I would continue losing weight.

Peter
Burroughs recommends drinking the Master Cleanse lemonade in the morning as a health regimen even after the cleanse. He also recommends a predominantly raw fruit, vegetable, seed, nut and berry diet.

Alternating one day each of a raw vegan diet and the Master Cleanse doesn't seem like a good idea to me. On the Master Cleanse, there is a detox day on about the seventh day. So staying on it for ten days makes a lot of sense to maximize the detoxifying effect.

As for the raw vegan diet, raw food author and lecturer, Victoria Boutenko, says it takes a week before the red blood cells recover from eating cooked food. In one of her recent lectures in Clearwater, Florida, she showed slides of red blood cells that were spherical and surrounded on all sides by plasma and then those taken one half hour after eating cooked food. In the latter slides, the red blood cells were all jammed together and no longer spherical. She said it takes a week for the red blood cells to return to their natural healthy shape. The maple syrup in the Master Cleanse is not considered a raw food.

So, although I have found both of these health regimens to be valuable, combining them *every other day* would seem to defeat the purpose of each. I recommend you do the Master Cleanse when you want, and otherwise eat the raw vegan diet or have the Master Cleanse lemonade in the morning.

Maple Syrup, Loving It a Little Too Much

Person No. 15
I've been measuring out my lemonades exactly (on Day 3 now) and am finding myself leaving a little extra maple syrup left over in the measuring spoon after I pour so that I can lick it up. Is this totally wrong, since I'm not supposed to be giving into cravings? Or is it alright since I was just going to consume that little bit anyway? Plus, I'm only using a tablespoon and a half versus two in each lemonade, and drinking only six to seven lemonades daily, because I know I have such a sweet tooth. Okay, I'm not alone here folks, right? Who else is loving the pure sugary organic goodness of their maple syrup as much as I?

Person No. 13
Once or twice a day I will eat a tablespoon of the maple syrup by itself. I don't see how this can be wrong, other than as extra calories if you are overweight, but I am losing weight anyway since I am still taking in less calories by far than I normally would. I don't think this would hurt anything at all. All the maple syrup is doing is providing you with nutrients anyway.

Person No. 15
Yeah, I thought so. Thanks. I have had the desire to just eat a tablespoon by itself once or twice.

Person No. 6
I'm on Day 9 and I found quite a few little things that I enjoy and consider treats during the cleanse. I feel so guilty posting this, but such is life. I like to do a teaspoon of pure maple syrup every now and then. The other day I did a couple of teaspoons of molasses, but that was too good. So I put the molasses away until after the cleanse. Did I cheat? No, I just made it fun for me. Please do not follow these terrible, disgusting little nuances because indeed they are habit forming. Good luck to all!

Person No. 15
Okay, we all must agree that it's not wrong and continue to find ways to enjoy ourselves during the cleanse. What else do we have?

Peter

I didn't say anything when you talked about sneaking a teaspoon here or there as it didn't sound like you were establishing new rules for the cleanse. However, when you said, "We all must agree that it's not wrong and continue to find ways to enjoy ourselves during the cleanse," I thought I had better speak up. You were probably just having fun and it was not your intention to change the rules, but we do not know how many other people will read this topic and change the actual directions. I would like to avoid that.

I don't think it's the end of the world or going to destroy all the benefits of the cleanse to have a little extra maple syrup once or twice on the entire cleanse. However, I would like to make it clear that the Master Cleanse as written by Stanley Burroughs does not include any extra maple syrup.

I've counseled or been aware of nearly a hundred cleanses by now and I know that if the cleanse directions are followed exactly a person will get the benefits that we are sharing on this bulletin board (provided the person is not on prescribed medications that prohibit the cleanse or that the person is not so toxic that cleansing is dangerous because it releases all those toxins too quickly.)

I am sorry if I sound like a strict school teacher, but I have already seen how changes in the successful directions sneak in with misconceptions and wanted to be sure that others get the benefits they seek.

As to having a craving for additional maple syrup, try increasing the amount in the drink to the full two tablespoons rather than eating the maple syrup separately. This will keep your blood sugar level more constant and reduce your craving for an extra teaspoon of maple syrup now and then.

Maple Syrup Substitute

Person No. 31

I have been drinking mint herbal tea. It is hard to drink without some kind of sweetener so I add Equal. Is there anything wrong with this?

● Peter

Regarding artificial sweeteners, I've heard Aspartame has been linked to some neurological degenerative diseases and may have something to do with fibromyalgia as well. Even after the cleanse, I'd recommend dropping them. As far as the cleanse is concerned, other than lemonade, salt water in the morning and laxative tea, plain mint tea is the only other thing mentioned by Stanley Burroughs in *The Master Cleanser*. I don't want to spoil your tea drinking, but while on the cleanse, you'll see more benefits if you stick to the cleanse as written.

Person No. 70

Hi all, great site. Can someone suggest a replacement for the maple syrup prescribed for the fast? I live in a smallish city in South Africa and absolutely cannot find maple syrup here at all. I'm afraid I've never seen any raw sugar cane stalks for sale anywhere. What do you think of using some other sweet juice as a last resort? I'm sure maple syrup would be best, but I guess we all have to do what we can. Many thanks.

Person No. 51

Possibly some pure, natural honey.

Person No. 13

No, honey (the book said) is to never be used as a substitute or internally ever. There is mention in the book about using a certain type of molasses (I think blackstrap) for people who are diabetic or can't use the maple syrup. Can you get molasses?

Person No. 52

Thanks for the tips. Yes, no problem getting blackstrap molasses. Do you know if the suggested use per glass of water is the same as maple syrup (two tablespoons)? Many thanks.

Person No. 13

Yes. It says for diabetics to work up to two tablespoons of blackstrap molasses. So hopefully this will work for you.

Maple Syrup, Unable to Handle the Taste of

Person No. 36

My wife started this with me and very quickly could not handle the taste of the maple syrup. She said if she had another glass with that aftertaste she would vomit. Is there an alternative she could use?

Peter

The only other thing Burroughs talks about is cane juice (notice, that's not cane syrup). My wife did it with soaked dates blended into date juice for about five days on her first cleanse. After that, she was able to handle the maple syrup. She got good results on date juice, but better results with maple syrup. If your wife does try date juice, please let us know how it goes. I'm always learning about the Master Cleanse.

Person No. 13

Make sure she is using organic grade B maple syrup as well, because the taste difference is just astounding between this and regular maple syrup. I had never tried organic grade B before and was amazed at the taste. My mother didn't want to try it either because she hates maple syrup, but when she did she said, "Wow! That is really good." I figure you're probably using the right thing, but just make sure because the taste difference is huge.

Person No. 43

Yeah, Person No.13 makes a great point here. Conventional methods for producing maple syrup include formaldehyde. This drastically reduces the taste and quality of maple syrup. I would suggest you make sure you have organic grade B maple syrup before you go out and buy cane juice.

Master Cleanse Beginner

Person No. 53

I like this forum because I can get in touch with others who are vegetarians, vegans, or raw foodists to decide what might be best for me.

I just started the cleanse yesterday and am very excited to see what happens. I have not read the book yet but plan to get it today. I was told about this cleanse by an acupuncturist. He told me I could have mint tea, is this true? Also, I didn't know I was supposed to start the cleanse with the salt water flush and I bought the wrong sea salt. It was iodized. So, I will get the right kind. I am so nervous doing this as I don't know the benefits, side effects, or even some of the smaller questions like, can I brush my teeth with toothpaste. I'm assuming not, so I haven't.

I have always been a healthy eater. However, for the last five months I was very bad and gained fifteen pounds. I am 5'2" and weigh 130. Will I lose healthy weight or muscle with the cleanse? Also, what do you think about the Blood Type Diet? I am a type B and have always eaten meat and dairy to keep down my weight. I've tried to be a vegetarian before and I gained weight. What do you suggest? I'm so sorry for all the questions. Your site is what has helped me so far and I really want to live healthily and inspire others with accurate information.

I couldn't do the salt water flush (SWF). It came back out. So, I bought Smooth Move (a laxative tea with senna and other herbs). Is this okay? My eliminations are mostly fluid. Is this normal? I don't know how I will be able to do the SWF as it makes me gag. Is there any other way? I have will power. However, once I drink it, it comes right back out! I really feel great already in three days. My skin is clearing up and I have a lot of energy! Hope to hear from you soon.

Peter
Stanley Burroughs recommends mint tea to help handle mouth and body odors because of its chlorophyll.

I'd recommend brushing your teeth with water only or bar soap and water and using the mint tea to freshen your mouth as quoted above.

Concerning losing healthy weight on the cleanse, Burroughs says the only thing you will lose is waste, not healthy tissue.

My personal opinion concerning eating protein and meat to keep weight off is that you are then eating too many acidic foods and throwing the body into an unhealthy situation. Burroughs promotes a raw fruit, nut and vegetable diet. So did Norman Walker, a naturopath who taught juicing and raw fruit and vegetable diets. He was active as a healer past the age of 100!

The salt water flush does indeed cause several eliminations within an hour or two (or longer for some people). The waste that is contained in the colon is impacted in layers and takes quite a while to detoxify and eliminate. Even though you are only seeing liquid (clear or yellow) for several days, you will pass some solid or semi-solid matter.

When I did a twenty-day Master Cleanse, I only passed solid waste on two or three days, but one of those was the seventeenth day. The "stuff" does indeed come off in layers and there's a lot there if you haven't done cleanses regularly for most of your life.

Is there another way? Yes. You can drink the laxative tea morning and night.

By the way, it is much easier to drink the salt water if you are using non-iodized sea salt rather than regular salt. My wife recommends using a straw if you want to avoid the super salty gag response. I've never needed to do that. So, I can't say if it works.

A senna blend tea such as Smooth Move is perfect, although all Burroughs says is "herb laxative tea."

That's great about your skin clearing up. The skin is one of the organs in the elimination system and in fact is the largest organ of the body. That it is clearing up means it is no longer overloaded with more toxic waste than it can handle.

Person No. 54
I have been using about three tablespoons of lemon juice with each glass for my own taste preference. I just read that you shouldn't alter the two tablespoons. Have I screwed up?

Peter
I doubt the extra lemon juice will ruin the cleanse. Whether it will yield the same excellent results is something I do not know. That is why I recommend following the Master Cleanse exactly as written. It works very well routinely.

If you want your lemonade less sweet, reduce the maple syrup. That is covered in the book.

Master Cleanse Book, Pass It Along

Person No. 55

Hi, all! I am brand spanking new. Heard about the Master Cleanse for the first time today. I am so excited to try this. I haven't gotten the book yet. I hope to get it tomorrow. I just have some quick questions. Can I have any herbal tea? Can I have chicken broth? Can I have V8 splash?

My friend did this with huge success. She wrote out an example day for me to follow:

Wake up: two glasses lemonade; Breakfast: herbal tea, lemonade; Snack: herbal tea, lemonade; Lunch: chicken broth; Snack: herbal tea, lemonade; Dinner: fresh fruit juice, lemonade; Snack: herbal tea, lemonade. So that's the day she gave me.

Is this ok? I'm afraid I won't have time to get the book tomorrow. I have a five-year-old and a six-month-old. I am not breast feeding and also work part-time in the evenings. I just don't want to start out doing the wrong thing.

This board is awesome and I am so excited I found it! If any of you could help me out, that would be so great. Thanks guys.

Peter

You will be surprised when you read the book because there is no chicken broth or fruit juice and your friend didn't mention the salt water flush in the morning.

I strongly recommend **everyone** who wants to do the Master Cleanse read the book. Verbal directions are like playing telephone, where you whisper something to someone who whispers what they heard to someone else, etc. down the line for five or ten people. The message is never the same.

I want you to get the best possible results. That will come by doing exactly what Stanley Burroughs developed. If you do not know what that is, you cannot be sure you are going to get the results you want.

Person No. 71

I read about this in a magazine and was intrigued. I looked it up on the web and started. I have never done a MC before. I have done a juice fast and detoxed other ways. I am excited about this, but I have two questions.

1. I did not read the book when beginning. The article I read said it was okay to have one twelve-ounce drink of organic fresh juice and one twelve-ounce bowl of fresh organic veggie broth. Is this okay or should I stop?

2. I have done the salt water internal bath. It worked well. That was a first. How many times should I do this? I am assuming from what I have read, every day?

Peter

1. Yes, you should stop drinking the fresh juice and veggie broth. The Master Cleanse as developed and written by Stanley Burroughs includes nothing but salt water in the a.m., six to twelve glasses daily of the lemon- or limeade, one cup of herbal laxative tea at night (and, optionally, one more in the morning), mint tea occasionally, and blackstrap molasses for diabetics during the cleanse. He does talk about slowly drinking several eight ounce glasses of fresh orange juice as desired throughout the day after completing the cleanse to break it. (Personally, I find the orange juice too heavy after the cleanse and prefer grapefruit juice.) He recommends a veggie broth soup as the evening meal on the second day after the cleanse. He gives a recipe for the soup in *The Master Cleanser* on page 26.

2. Yes, the salt water flush is done each morning of the cleanse. The worksheet on www.TheMasterCleanse.com (and earlier in this book) gives you the items and the times to use them.

You should also be drinking the herbal laxative tea each evening as you'll see on the worksheet. By the way, the worksheet is *not* meant to replace the book. The book has lots of other valuable information.

Person No. 16

I am in high school. I get up at 5:00 in the morning and leave the house at 6:10, I can't do the salt in the morning because I don't think I will have enough time to let it work. Can I do the salt flush when I come home, usually 3:30 p.m., but some days at 5:30? I know you said not to flush so that the lemonade and pepper can work overnight, but I don't have any of the pepper! Don't you think the flush will work and be done at 5:00? I also wanted to know if sarsaparilla tea is good enough.

Peter

That is great that you are taking such good care of your body at your age. If you cannot do the flush, drink the herb laxative tea night and morning like the book says.

You must go to the store and buy some cayenne pepper. It is sold as red pepper. It helps to dissolve the mucus and build the blood. It also opens the blood vessels to increase the flow of nutrients to the body's cells. It's not the Master Cleanse without it. It is quite inexpensive.

Sarsaparilla tea is not a laxative. Herbal references say that sarsaparilla is good for gout and rheumatism and is very similar to testosterone in the body, but it is not a laxative. Licorice root is a mild laxative. Senna is a stronger one. Go to the health food store and buy a combination tea with both of those in it.

Please buy the book and read it. It sounds like you're missing the mark with no salt water, no cayenne and drinking sarsaparilla tea. I want you to get all the benefits you can.

Please, when you care enough about others' health to tell them about the Master Cleanse, please care enough to see they read the book. Give it to them, send them to www.TheMasterCleanse.com, or send them to a store to buy it. It only costs $6.50. From the above postings to the bulletin board, you can see the misinformation that gets passed on when the book is not used as the source of how to do the Master Cleanse.

Medication

Person No. 56

I take Wellbutrin for minimal depression. Should I still take it or discontinue it for the fast?

Peter

I'm not a medical doctor and even if I were, I don't have your complete medical history, chart and any diagnostic test results. So, I would not even dream of advising you as to whether you should discontinue your medicine. You should seek the advice of your licensed health care provider and use your own good judgment.

Here is some information that you may find useful to help make your decision.

1. The purpose of a cleanse is to remove toxins and old waste from the body. The body in most cases treats medical drugs as toxins from a digestive standpoint. So, putting more in while trying to get toxins out doesn't make a lot of sense. Thus, any **non-essential** medicines, i.e. allergy medicines, that are not necessary for maintaining life, might best be omitted.

2. Occasionally, the body stores some of the medicine it is taking. I have heard that one or two full doses of strong anti-depressant or chemotherapy medicines may be stored in the body and could possibly be released on a cleanse. So, if you do decide to do the cleanse, have taken strong medicine, and begin to feel the effects of a dose or two of your old medicine, I advise ending the cleanse and instead doing a much gentler and slower detox such as with herbs and bentonite clay or just a raw food diet with juicing (*not* juicing alone). You can always come back to the Master Cleanse again later after you have done a slower form of detox.

3. Another alternative is to discontinue **non-essential** medication, such as diet or sleeping pills that were not prescribed by a licensed health care professional, for a while before the cleanse. This way, you can be stable without the medication before starting the cleanse. **If you are on a prescribed medication, especially such as that to avoid a heart attack, stroke or other fatal event, do *not* discontinue your medicine without consulting the prescribing licensed health care practitioner!**

5. As far as doing the cleanse while being on the medication, in a recent survey of 137 people who have done or are doing the Master Cleanse, only one person reported having any problems at all with their medication. And that lady only had problems one of the ten times she had done the cleanse.

I'm sorry I can't give you a yes or no answer, but I hope this helps.

Person No. 72
Peter, I read your article in *Natural Awakenings*, researched the Master Cleanse on the web, and went to your website as mentioned in the article. Thanks for providing this website. It was a great blessing to me, a first time MCer. In fact, my mother, seventy-one years old, and my brother, forty-three years old, and sister, thirty years old, will be doing the MC for the first time starting in February.

My mother is on medication. She takes blood pressure and blood thinning medications. I told her to do the MC gradually, in small time allocations (this first time she is only doing a thirty-six-hour cleanse), then listen to her body and see how she feels. She has a doctor's appointment scheduled a day after she breaks her fast. Her goal is to be able to do a thirty-six-hour fast once a month for a while, then progress to a three-day fast, then a five-day fast, etc. until her health will allow her to complete the minimum ten-day fast in the future, perhaps next year this time.

Peter
The one person I know who had high blood pressure going into the cleanse noticeably reduced it on the cleanse and kept it lower (although not as low as while on the cleanse) with a raw vegetarian diet.

Be sure to run the concept of the cleanse lowering blood pressure by her doctor for coordination purposes and to make sure she doesn't get a double whammy from the combined effects of the medication and the cleanse and faint when she stands up. Be sure she knows to stand up slowly and have someone watch her.

I think your idea of short cleanses until she's stable is a good idea.

I think the blood thinning is also handled by a raw vegetarian diet, but don't have any experience or facts.

● Person No. 72
Thanks for your response. My mom is so excited. She will actually start the thirty-six-hour Master Cleanse Monday, Feb. 2, 2004. After that, depending on how she feels she may extend the cleanse a few more days. I will keep a close eye on her and cheer her on when she starts getting detox symptoms and will want to quit. She has been using medications for years. We will take it slow.

Regarding her blood pressure medication, the doctor has scheduled her every three months, the first appointment the first Friday in February, to monitor it in order to reduce the dose as required. I think the MC is the best thing that ever happened to her and me for that matter. I enlighten everyone that I come in contact with.

Thanks again Peter. May God bless you and your entire family!

Person No. 54
I have been on a low dose of Zoloft for the past three years. I am continuing to take it. I'm on Day 5. Will it somehow interfere with the cleanse?

Peter
See my reply at the beginning of this topic to Person No. 56. In addition, I recommend the book, *Potatoes, not Prozac* by Kathleen DesMaisons (available at www.TheMasterCleanse.com). It explains how a proper diet can address mental distress that is actually caused by the wrong diet.

Minerals

Person No. 49
I currently take all natural liquid magnesium chloride. I know that the maple syrup has some magnesium, but wanted to know if it would be okay to take the liquid magnesium (one-half teaspoon) with the drink. It is not a pill, therefore it would not need to be as digested as a pill would, correct?

Peter
The lemon provides magnesium. It acts as a blood alkalizer. I recommend you follow the cleanse as written and abstain from any supplements until after the cleanse. *The Master Cleanser* says you do not need and should not take any supplements while on the cleanse.

Mucoid Plaque

[Mucoid plaque is a tough rubbery coating that forms from mucus and accumulated waste on the large intestine walls. There are numerous pictures of this on the Web.]

Person No. 13

I want to see this [referring to a picture on the web] come out of me, more than anything. How many people here have shed mucoid? I saw that one person did, on another topic. Should I expect to definitely see this happen if I stay on the fast for about twenty days? Or, do you think it comes out regardless on the cleanse, maybe just not all in one piece like that?

Person No. 12

Hey girl, I have not seen that yet and I am on Day 4. If that's what's inside me, I'll be happy when I see it come out! GOOD LAWD! That must be a scary sight!

Person No. 11

I am on Day 9 and I haven't seen that horror yet!

Person No. 13

Well, that usually comes from doing a typical colon cleanse with lots of supplements and colonics. But, I am hoping this cleanse will get rid of it just as well. Maybe it just doesn't take that form. Maybe it just comes out in smaller pieces instead of all at once, like I said. I hope so. Anyone else with feedback about this, please reply.

Peter

I've only heard of one person who described an elimination that could have been mucoid plaque and that person fit the description of someone who ate the SAD diet and had never done a cleanse, colonic, nor eaten a raw food diet.

Most times, the accumulated waste is just dissolved over several days by the lemon juice and cayenne, washed by the salt water, and broken up into small mucousy flakes by the increased intestinal action brought on by the herbal laxative tea. That's always been the case for me. Even after seventeen days of not eating, I've had mucousy flakes eliminated.

I think anyone wanting to see foot-long sections (or longer) of mucoid plaque needs to go on a water fast with colonics rather than the Master Cleanse. Personally, I prefer the Master Cleanse.

Person No. 13

Well, I was hoping that it just got broken into pieces. I don't care how it comes out, just as long as it does. I would much rather have it come out gradually than have to sit on the toilet for hours and have it all come out in one big piece like it does with a traditional colon cleanse. I'm not patient enough for that.

Nothing Happening

Person No. 12
I am on Day 5. No solid bowel movement, no weight loss, no increase in energy. The only thing is that I'm not groggy in the morning and have weird dreams! That's it. I'm going to continue and not give up, but I am getting frustrated. My girlfriend lost nine pounds in the first four days. Ugh!

Peter
Well, let's look at all the points where this cleanse could go wrong and see if we can sort it out.

1. Are you putting two teaspoons of non-iodized sea salt in the salt water each morning and drinking it as fast as possible?

2. Are you mixing two tablespoons (one ounce) of fresh squeezed — not bottled — lemon juice into each ten-ounce drink or using these proportions for each batch and no more than one day's worth at a time?

3. Are you putting in an increasing amount of cayenne pepper to taste with each drink?

4. Are you drinking one cup of laxative tea each morning as well as each evening to encourage more elimination?

5. Are you eating or drinking anything else but water and occasional mint tea?

6. Before this cleanse, did you have only one or two BMs per week? Being constipated before the cleanse might mean a little longer before you'd see results.

7. Are you on any constipating medications? I'm NOT suggesting you come off any prescribed medications. Just that they may alter the results of the cleanse.

Person No. 12

Peter, Thanks for the input. You helped me out a LOT. Ok here are my faults:

1) On Days 1-4 I had been using two tablespoons of salt, not teaspoons. I used two teaspoons today (Day 5) and it has not come out yet.

2) I am using an herbal tea only at night, NOT MORN—I will increase that to a morning cup.

3) I've always been a once a day bathroom girl, so I think it may take longer for me.

4) I am using a laxative herbal tea with senna, but not Smooth Move. The one I've been using contains other herbs as well as added vitamins (I think vitamin C). I will switch teas to Smooth Move and start taking one cup at night and in the morning.

I can say I am doing the drink correctly. I measure my lemonade drinks perfectly and I use organic lemons and maple syrup with plenty of cayenne. I usually drink six to ten glasses a day and about sixty-four to ninety-six ounces of water in between!

My only other concern—I use Crystal Springs Mountain bottled water from the store. Is this ok?

Peter

The bottled water is okay so long as it does not contain fluoride.

The only other thought I have for you or any others not seeing results by Day 5 is that some people who have lived on the SAD diet (Standard American Diet) and are overweight may take a while before enough accumulated waste is loosened and eliminated to start seeing results. I'd say go for the full ten days. That's what Burroughs says.

Person No. 16

I suggest Yellow Dock tea because it is just as effective as any senna blend and it is fast acting, painless and smooth, whereas senna can cause intestinal spasms.

If you're worried about taste though, don't use Yellow Dock because it tastes literally like the bark of a tree. But I kind of like that because I'm a very strict vegan/raw vegan and I like to taste pure nature. Good luck!!

For the first few days, I had no bowel movements. However, I just added a little more tea to my water and now I make a few. I am losing weight, too. I'm on the sixth day and I've lost nine pounds.

Since I'm writing a comment here, I might as well ask my question: I know that in the book Burroughs says that fatty tissue melts away and is eliminated, but another place in the book he says nothing but toxins and diseases are eliminated, so I just wanted to know if some of the weight I'm losing is actual.

Peter

Toxins are stored in the fat. This is one of the reasons for so many overweight Americans. It is the result of their SAD diet. The preservatives, artificial colors and flavors and other non-real-food that they eat are treated by the body as toxins. What it cannot eliminate, it stores in fat cells. Lose the toxins...lose the fat!

Person No. 16

What about this quote on page thirteen, "As a reducing diet it is superior in every way to any other system because it dissolves and eliminates all types of fatty tissue. Fat melts away at the rate of about two pounds a day for most persons—and without any harmful side effects."

Peter

When you release the toxins with the cleanse or eating only a raw vegetarian diet, the fat is no longer needed as the toxins are gone and the body sheds the fat.

Person No. 17

I'm on the end of Day 4, but don't feel like I am gaining a lot more energy, losing any weight or having any real positive results. I know I am detoxing based on the last two days. I felt good the first two days and Day 3 was weird. I had mild tingling sensations in different body parts, a jaw ache, a mild sore throat, a groggy brain and food cravings. Today was just the worst, only because I wanted to eat sooooo bad. Everything looked good.

My BMs seem normal, getting some waste out each morning. I am doing everything (almost) as prescribed in the book, laxative tea at

116

night, salt water flush in the morning, but here is my concern. I can barely manage to get down six cups of lemonade a day. (Some days it has been five and one-quarter). When I do finish a cup I notice a lot of the pepper seems to be left at the bottom and I do not drink the pepper-filled last ounce in the cup. Yuck!

In fact, I cheat a bit on the pepper because it tastes so bad and only put in 1/16 tsp. instead of the prescribed 1/10th. After all, who has a 1/10 measuring spoon? This has to be a bit of a guess for most doesn't it? (Don't advise the cayenne pills, I don't swallow pills well.)

Anyway, I wonder how just barely drinking the minimum affects the cleanse and is using just slightly less pepper a big deal? Does it stand to reason that if you are a small person it would be sufficient to drink less than if you weighed a 100 lbs. more? Just a hopeful thought.

If anyone has any comments on how they manage to get in seven or more cups I would love to hear.

Thanks for reading this lengthy message. Reading all of your messages has given me some encouragement at a time when I really need it.

Peter
Hi Person No.17, those are good questions.

One way to get down more lemonade is to drink only lemonade until you reach your quota. Drink your first glass about one-half to one hour after the salt water. Then drink a glass every hour. This will make you pee frequently. Every time you pee, drink another glass. (This is what my wife recommends.)

On the cayenne, it speeds everything up. It dilates blood vessels, breaks up the mucus and increases circulation and metabolism. You are quite correct: it is all estimation regarding measuring the cayenne. Do not put so much in that you hate the taste of the lemonade and then can't drink it. However, do try to stretch your tolerance of it.

It is important to mix up the lemonade just before you drink it, so you get the cayenne. Not getting enough cayenne will definitely slow down your cleanse. I mix up the cayenne by making up four drinks at a time in a large plastic bottle and shaking the bottle every time just before I drink it.

The other thing to understand is that this is a ten-day process. Yes, some people get results more quickly than others, but do not judge your results by what happens after five, six or seven days. My wife learned that there were many days when she did not lose pounds, but then she discovered that she was losing inches. Her body was changing shape for the better rather than losing weight.

Take a longer view. If you get enough lemonade and cayenne, you'll not be straining to try to make it to Day 6. You'll be cruising with the rest of us.

By the way, the minimum for smaller people is six drinks per day, not seven. Hope this helps.

Person No. 13

If all else fails, hold your nose and chug! I started doing this when I started drinking green veggie juice (kale, collard, cucumber, celery) which tastes awful, but is awesome for you. It also helps to think of what you're taking as medicine, because it is—just like when you were a child and would hold your nose for medicine. Think of it the same way and this doesn't taste nearly as bad as most of that stuff.

As far as the pepper goes, just mix it up really well, and chug, chug, chug, even if you have trouble doing this at first. Your breathing and throat will adjust so that you can.

Person No. 17

Peter and Person No.13, thank you both for your responses. Today was a better day. I quit drinking the lemonade in a cup and have switched to a bottle with a straw and that seems to help me drink it faster. I might try the nose-holding thing if I really want to chug. But the pepper burns my throat and makes me cough sometimes.

Well, finishing Day 5 makes me feel like I am over the hump. It can only get better from here, right? Thanks for the ideas and encouragement. I appreciate it.

Person No. 47

I'm on Day 5 of the MC. Have been doing it just as the book says—the salt water every morning, lemonade during the day, and Smooth Move tea at night. I have a few questions about what is supposed to be happening now.

1) I wonder if I'm eliminating toxins or not. The only thing coming out now is a bright yellow liquid. Also, my tongue is pink. It got a yellowish coating for the first two days, but has since looked pink and normal.

2) I am sick of drinking lemonade. For the past two days, I've only had four cups a day instead of the minimum six. How important is it to keep up the six-drink minimum?

3) In the first three days, I dropped about six pounds, but since then I have not seen additional weight loss. I feel as though I'm at a standstill right now.

I would like to keep going but it's getting harder now that I'm feeling like I've hit a plateau. Thanks for your help!

● Peter

Lots of people wonder if they're eliminating toxins or not. The waste comes off in layers. So, you don't see anything happening for days and then have a detox day and see some results. I'd encourage you to continue through the ten days. When I did my first cleanse (twenty days) I had bright yellow liquid for about a week in the middle of the twenty days. Then I had some semi-solid waste and felt great the next day.

If you don't drink the minimum, you won't detox as much. Lots of fluids help to cleanse the kidneys and liver as well as the colon.

My wife discovered that just weighing yourself is not a good measure because she found that her body was changing shape and losing inches even when she was not losing weight.

Your statement, "I would like to keep going but it's getting harder now that I'm feeling like I've hit a plateau," sounds like a detox day. Let us know how you feel tomorrow.

Person No. 57

I am in my third day of my fast but I feel like I am doing something wrong because I am not seeing much of a change. I decided to go on the fast because I plan on becoming a vegan and wanted to start my new way of life with a cleansed body. The problems that led me to becoming a vegan are my eczema, stomach problems, and back pains. During my fast so far, my stomach has not really hurt. I only feel discomfort right before a bowel movement. Unfortunately, I am still having back pains and I am still scratching my itchy skin. I thought maybe the pain was heightened from all the toxins moving around in my body but I am not sure. The reason I am unsure is because of my BMs.

I apologize if this is TMI (too much information) but I need some help in understanding what is happening to my body. On the first day of my fast, my BM was solid and then runny. On the second and now third I go to the bathroom at least three times, but my BM is small and runny. I don't know if it is because that's all that is in my body. But I think that is not the case because my eczema and back are still acting up. I think I am clogged up and I wanted to know what I could do to clear my system.

I tried drinking the salt water flush but I could not manage it and I am drinking the herbal tea at night and in the morning. Should I try two cups of tea and can I try using one tablespoon of salt in the flush so I can keep it down? Any advice would be appreciated. Thank you.

● Peter

Many, myself among them, think the Master Cleanse is the ideal way to begin a move to a healthier diet (only raw fruits, vegetables, nuts and seeds being very, very healthy) as it removes cravings for the processed and cooked foods when it removes the toxins. (See the topic above "Detox Symptoms—Don't Hate Them: They Are Milestones.")

Concerning your situation, the third day is probably too soon to notice big changes if you've never done a cleanse and have been eating meat and cheese most of your life. Big changes usually come after Day 7.

Next, it does sound like you need the salt water flush as well as the tea to move things along. Generally, if you feel like you're clogged up, you probably are. Be sure you're using thirty-two ounces of water and non-iodized sea salt. Then be sure you're only using level teaspoons, not tablespoons. Then try drinking it through a straw. If all that fails, then try your idea of lessening the amount of salt, but don't go all the way down to one teaspoon.

The reason for the salt is to make the density (scientifically, the specific gravity—this is explained in Part II) of the water match that of blood so that the kidneys don't absorb the water and the blood doesn't absorb the salt. Then all of it can wash through the system in a dramatic way.

Some people have to drink a few days of salt water before they see a result, so stick with it.

If you have any other questions, just ask. This is a cleanse and the purpose is to eliminate. So these questions about BMs have to be asked and answered so the benefits can be had.

Just continue. It will come out okay in the end.

Person No. 8

Having done the Master Cleanse once before, I can really say that I feel doing the whole thirty-two ounces of salt water is very important. It does get easier the more your drink it. I can down the whole thing in two minutes, although, when I first get up in the morning the thought of doing it is enough to make me want to go back to bed.

I first got in touch with Peter when I did the first cleanse. I had stopped doing the salt water because I didn't feel it was doing me any good. It just ran right out of me. Peter explained that it is supposed to do that to clean the colon walls. I started doing the salt water again on that cleanse. After being on the cleanse already for a few days, I was surprised as to how much came out. This is after me being on a 90% raw food diet (with occasional cheating when going out to a restaurant). So what I am saying is my colon was pretty well cleaned out to begin with.

Over the holidays I ate junk stuff and a little meat and cheese. That food over the six-week period caused my bowels not to move as often as when I got off of the cleanse in November. You should be having a bowel movement after every meal and I was at first. Now on Day 5 of the cleanse my stomach is flat because my colon is really getting cleaned out and I will continue doing the flush after the cleanse because I feel it is very important to keep the colon clean.

A clogged colon is the root of all diseases. If you have never done anything to clean your colon, think about a dirty floor with years of built-up dirt. If you wiped it down you would only get the top layer of dirt so you would have to keep cleaning it. I have been on the Hallelujah Diet since September 2002, and gradually switched to mostly raw this past summer, but it wasn't until I did the Master Cleanse the first time that I felt like my colon was really clean. I had also done several other colon cleansing methods. The Master Cleanse is the quickest, cheapest way to go. Good luck.

Person No. 57

Thank you very much for the response and advice. I will try doing the salt water flush again tomorrow morning. It is Day 4 and I am feeling optimistic. Thanks again.

Person No. 2

I agree with the comments about the salt water flush. Yes, it sucks. Yes, it is awful. Yes, you feel like there is nothing worse you can do to yourself. However, within an hour I have an elimination. That says this stuff works.

I am on my second Master Cleanse. On the first one, I had solid BMs through Day 8. My wife, an RN, didn't believe me. I offered to keep the stuff in the bowl for her to review (joke). She became a believer.

This time (second Master Cleanse) I had one solid BM on Day 3 and one on Day 9. Other than that it looked like salt water mixed with the lemonade. The floor analogy above is a good one. This stuff is coming off/out in layers.

Peter told me that when he eats food that is not good for him, he downs the salt water flush the next morning. I tried that after a red meat day with cheese. For me, it is two or three flushes to get back to feeling good.

Person No.57, I hope you can do the salt water. I think that and a couple of days will start giving you some very tangible signs of improvement. Good luck.

Pain

Person No. 13

Okay, this is my second day on the fast and I am in terrible pain. I'm trying to figure out why and if I will be able to stay on the fast. I really want to.

Yesterday I had a couple of fairly large eliminations. I know this is stuff that's been trapped in there a while. Because of my raw diet I am able to tell what exactly is coming out of me, and this was unrecognizable.

The first one like this was okay. The second one was in the middle of the night last night and I woke up in extreme pain, sweats, etc. After I used the restroom I was able to go back to sleep, but my stomach hurt a while before I could.

Today has been awful. Very, very bad stomach pain and burning. It feels like a lot of stomach acid. I'm familiar with this feeling because my stomach used to overproduce acid. Before I changed my diet, my pH was very bad and my stomach would hurt this way often—just not this badly.

Today I am eliminating a lot of bile and just a little bit of other stuff. The pain seems to subside after I eliminate for a little while, but then it comes right back. I have been too ill to even drink anything yet today, but I am about to try.

I was wondering if anyone has any suggestions on how to combat this horrible pain, if someone else went through the same thing at first, and if it subsided, approximately when. I know it will vary a bit from person to person, but I need some reassurance and to see if this is normal. As much as I want and need to do this fast, I will not be able to if this doesn't start going away. I'm barely able to sit up straight right now and it's definitely interfering with my ability to work. Any suggestions/relative stories would be appreciated.

Person No.13 [This was a later addition.]
I just read the topic about detox symptoms and how the nausea, etc., only occurs if you're extremely toxic. I have no doubt that, despite my good eating habits over the past year, I still have a lot of toxic buildup, which is why I'm doing the fast. I will try to stick it out for at least a few days and hope this subsides, as suggested in the detox topic. Still, if anyone else has experienced stuff like this I would appreciate the encouragement.

Person No. 11
Hang in there. I was actually having those symptoms on Days 7 and 8. I don't think it was the senna tea because I was fine with it for the first six days. However, I did experience intense abdominal pain. It felt like something was bubbling in there and I had quite a bit of pain when it was time to eliminate. I also experienced the burning and I could only attribute it to the cayenne since I am eating nothing else! Don't forget that you will have those painful days that normally resolve

themselves within the next couple of days. Be sure to drink lots of water. I didn't really drink much because I was so bloated with the lemonade, but now I am making the effort to add extra water. I suppose this first cleanse is a learning period for me. I know for a fact that this will be a lot easier the second time, so hang in there and lots of luck!

● Peter

Let's see if we can sort out the pain. Pure senna tea can be too strong and cause a cramping feeling in the abdomen which goes away once the salt water is drunk or lots of lemonade. If that is the case, switch to an herb blend that has senna and other ingredients. Try Smooth Move or Get Regular. Drink it only the last thing at night just before you go to sleep. It should take six to twelve hours before it causes eliminations. Sometimes it's faster. That way your eliminations will be right when you wake up in the morning instead of in the middle of the night.

Interestingly, on my first cleanse, I had very burning BMs from Days 2–7. They do go away. One thing you can do to handle this is drink lots of liquids. Toxins are acidic and apparently you have a lot of them ready to be eliminated. As you continue the cleanse, the lemonade will dissolve these and the BMs will get easier.

Have you taken a lot of medications? Are you overweight? Do you have allergies? All of these are indications of toxicity. More toxicity means the harder the first few days will be relative to others who aren't in that condition. Either way, it gets much easier after Day 5.

Your best course of action is to emphasize the elimination side of the cleanse with drinking lots of lemonade, water, the standard amount of laxative tea and the salt water flush. If it gets to be too much, end the cleanse for now, clean up your diet and do the cleanse again. Remember, getting healthy is not a one-time event. It's a lifetime process.

Person No. 13

Well, as long as I know that it can be normal to have that much pain, I will keep on the cleanse. I am very stubborn. As far as cleaning up my diet goes, I don't think I could possibly clean it up any more. I have been a raw vegan since last June and before that I was a vegan for a couple of months. Now, I realize that the longer I am raw, the better I will feel, but I don't think I can ever reap the full benefits of the lifestyle without doing a cleanse, which is why I am doing one now. Obviously, I have a lot to clean out.

Why? Well, not only did I eat the SAD for 22 years, but worse than that, I am from Louisiana and so therefore I ate the VERY SAD, the Southern American Diet. I ate lots of fried fatty foods, little to no veggies (and those were always cooked and smothered in butter/sugar/you name it), not to mention that I drank nothing but Coke most of my life, tap water when I did have water, used ephedra pills for two years, and did the Atkins diet for a year. Our air quality is very poor. I have breathed in a ton of secondhand smoke. I was never properly fed as a child as my parents never made me eat raw fruits or vegetables and I did not have proper exercise.

All this led to a super case of fibromyalgia which I have had symptoms of since I was about eleven. But at this point I understand it to basically be malnutrition and very bad body pH. I have pretty much conquered it through being raw and juicing greens every day to keep my vitamins and nutrients up and my pH alkaline. The changes have been really amazing and it's really such a simple concept. I wish more people were better educated on these things and willing to make the changes to get healthier.

As far as being overweight, I am 5' 2" and 115 lbs. For myself, (I wish to be 10% body fat or less) I probably still have fifteen to twenty pounds of fat to lose. I do have a lot of body fat, no doubt there. All these things would be a good explanation as to why I am so toxic. I anticipate getting rid of it. I'll do anything to be healthier and continue on this path. I will not stop. Thanks for your support.

Parasites

Person No. 13
Anyone seen any wormy friends come out? Because I swear I just flushed about three of them.

Peter
This cleanse definitely gets rid of them. I've read that one of the signs of parasites is picking the nose. (Yes, it's that common.) After about five days on the cleanse, my nose picking stopped. It doesn't come back as long as I don't eat meat. Once I start on ribs (my favorite) or other types of meat, I start again. The parasites need accumulated acid waste matter to survive. A clean, healthy bowel will not support them.

This is just another bonus of the Master Cleanse.

Personal Health, Observations on

Peter

1. Each person is responsible for his or her own health.

2. It is wise for a person to learn how to maintain and/or improve their health.

3. Valuable knowledge is available if you take the time to look for it and are willing to determine for yourself whether any knowledge presented is true or false.

4. Each person's body is potentially different. For example, most people find penicillin valuable for killing bacteria. Some people are allergic and die from it.

5. Diagnosis or advice from a health professional is frequently essential, but each person is responsible to determine if it is true or not for his or her own body and whether to follow the treatment.

6. You should use your own good judgment and experience in determining whether to apply the knowledge offered in this book or on the bulletin board at www.TheMasterCleanse.com. Do not accept it blindly. This may mean consulting a health professional.

Pregnant, Trying to Get

Person No. 12

I've been spotting the whole cleanse. I have had problems getting pregnant, so I think my uterine and girlie organs are repairing themselves. I had a miscarriage last year. I was not producing some hormone that is supposed to double when you're pregnant. Luckily, I lost the baby in the first month. Now the doctor wants to put me on some pills to help me ovulate more. I don't believe ovulating is my problem. I think it's deeper than that. I have been unhealthy for a long time and I think my body can repair itself with this cleanse. I am going to wait to let God do his work. I am going to try for two more months after this cleanse to get pregnant. I'll keep you posted in the months to come.

Peter

I recommend two books: *The Wheatgrass Book* by Ann Wigmore, and *Grower Younger* by Norman Walker. Both are natural, nutritional methods to improve the general health of the body.

Person No. 54

I'm on Day 5. This is the second time I've done the cleanse.

My husband and I had been trying to get pregnant for two years. In August of 2002, I quit smoking, then did the five-day MC in September. Lo and behold, in October I discovered I was pregnant. Just an interesting note. The second time is easier, and I'm ready to ride it out until the ole tongue turns pink again, even if that means going beyond ten days. I feel very fortunate that I stumbled on your site. Thanks.

Peter

This is long, but well worth reading and explains why I gave the references above. It is a synopsis of "Pottenger's Cats — A Study in Nutrition," by Francis M. Pottenger, Jr., MD.

From 1932 to 1942, Dr. Francis Marion Pottenger, Jr. conducted an experiment on the effects of heat-processed food on cats.

Dr. Pottenger had an adrenal extract manufacturing company in southern California. At that time, there were no chemical procedures to measure the strength of adrenal extract. So, manufacturers used cats. Cats die without their adrenal glands. So, the amount of extract the cats needed to keep them alive allowed the manufacturers to calibrate the strength of their product. His interest was prompted by the high death rate among his laboratory cats undergoing operations to remove their adrenal glands.

The cats were fed a diet of raw milk, cod liver oil and cooked meat scraps because this was considered the best diet for cats at the time. Concerned with the cats' general health and postoperative survival, Dr. Pottenger noticed the cats had decreased reproductive capacity and that many of their kittens had skeletal deformities and organ malfunctions.

Since this was the middle of the Great Depression and since his neighbors in Monrovia kept sending him increasing numbers of cats they couldn't or didn't want to feed, he couldn't handle the demand for cooked meat scraps. So he ordered raw meat scraps from a local meat packing plant. Always a scientist, Dr. Pottenger fed the raw meat scraps to a separate group of cats so that he could observe any differences between the groups of cats. Within a few months, this group was healthier, their kittens more vigorous, and they had a higher survival rate after their operations.

The contrast between the two sets of cats was so striking, Dr. Pottenger decided to perform a scientific experiment to verify these differences.

The experiment included 900 cats over four generations. The cats were divided into five groups. Each group was supplied with the same basic diet requirements, except for the staple (major part) of the diet. Each group received one of the following staples: raw milk, raw meat scraps, pasteurized milk, evaporated milk or condensed milk.

The raw meat and raw milk groups remained healthy throughout their normal lifespan through all four generations. The first generation of all three processed food groups developed diseases and illnesses near the end of their lives. The second generation of the three processed food groups developed diseases and illnesses in the middle of their lives. The third generation of all three processed food groups developed diseases and illnesses in the beginning of their lives and many died before six months of age. There was no fourth generation in any of the three processed food groups! Either the third generation parents were sterile or the fourth generation cats died before birth. Remember, all four generations of the raw food groups were healthy throughout their normal lifespan.

Is this why so many children are now developing cancer? Why there were no fertility clinics thirty years ago?

There has been no similar experiment ever conducted in scientific literature. The findings were supervised by Dr. Pottenger along with a professor of pathology at the University of Southern California, who was also a pathologist at the Huntington Memorial Hospital in Pasadena.

[This information is based on a report published by the Price-Pottenger Nutrition Foundation, www.price-pottenger.org, which sells copies of the book containing this report.]

Protein—a Raw Vegetarian Diet and Weight Lifting

Person No. 1

I am new to the MC way of life. I was curious as to what effect the MC and Stanley Burroughs' recommended nutritional diet would have on a person who lifts weights since Mr. Burroughs' ideas regarding consuming meat for protein are not positive.

Before starting the MC, I ate meat (chicken or fish) once a day and the rest of my meals consisted of raw or steamed veggies and fruit. I would obtain the rest of my daily protein requirement by using protein powders mixed in water. I always ate a balanced protein/carbohydrate/fat ratio as recommended by Bill Phillips (*Body for Life*). That seems to work for me in balancing my hormones, food cravings and weight control/management.

Question: If I need protein to help repair the muscle I tear down during a lifting session, where am I going to get the needed protein if I am only eating raw/steamed fruits and veggies? (Dairy products are no answer for me as I am lactose intolerant.)

Peter

I am not familiar with Bill Phillips' program, but I can tell you what I have learned about the Master Cleanse and a raw fruit/vegetable/nut/seed diet.

Spirulina has more than 60% protein by weight compared to beef or chicken, which have about 20%. (Sunflower seeds and almonds also have about 20% by the way.) Eggs have less than 5%, about the same as broccoli and cauliflower. (SOURCE: Paul Pitchford, *Healing with Whole Foods*, p.143)

In *The Wheatgrass Book* by Ann Wigmore, she talks about a raw fruit/vegetable/nut/seed diet along with wheatgrass juice as supplying all the needed protein and other nutrients to rebuild the body. Remember, the largest land animals are vegetarians. They have no trouble building huge muscular bodies with protein. If you feel you need more protein, start adding soaked almonds and seeds to your diet as well. (Soaking the seeds and nuts releases the enzyme inhibiter—the substance that keeps them from sprouting—and makes them easier to digest.)

Victoria and Igor Boutenko, authors of the *Raw Family*, spoke a few weeks ago in our area. They said they have seen people lose weight when they first go on an all raw diet and then their bodies rebuild to a healthy weight after some time.

Igor talked about being able to do *hundreds* of pushups at a time as a result of the body he's rebuilt over many years as a 100% raw vegetarian.

Running or Exercising During the Diet

Person No. 73
I run approximately fifteen miles per week. Will I need to lay off the running during the cleanse?

Peter
Everyone I know who has done the cleanse has had increased energy. People who do water fasts need bed rest, but not Master Cleansers.

Indeed, I have a friend that runs five miles nearly every day. When he went on a water fast, he had to give up running and could only walk by the fifth day. On the Master Cleanse, he was running all the way up to the twentieth day when he finished the cleanse. Another friend was used to walking four miles a day. On the cleanse he started walking six miles a day and occasionally running a few miles as well! These are not unusual cases. Nearly everyone is surprised to find they have noticeably more energy.

You may occasionally have what I call detox days (usually the second, third, seventh and fifteenth—if you go that long) where you feel tired, irritable or want to eat something solid. However, the symptoms usually pass in a day or two and you feel even better afterward.

Person No. 17
I just want to confirm what Peter said. I work out regularly at the gym. I do one hour on the elliptical machine, which is about five miles. I did this workout with lots of energy on Day 6 of the cleanse.

Also, I provide Swedish massage for a living and on Day 2 I gave three one-hour massages and one hour-and-a-half massage back to back, which is quite a workout and normally would make me quite tired. I felt great afterwards. Again, on Day 5, I did four one-hour massages back to back with lots of energy. I have had much more energy on the MC and without any dips or lows like I usually do at 3:00 p.m. I think you'll find your workout will be no problem and perhaps even better. Good luck!

Person No. 31

I'm on Day 2. At noon, I went to the gym to do my normal routine. I run three miles, do 100 crunches, some arm curls, etc. and had plenty of energy. Overall, I feel great.

Salt Water Flush

Peter

Others I've talked to have occasionally found that the first day or two of drinking the salt water didn't produce any elimination. Usually this is true of those who eat meat or dairy products regularly. Adjusting the salt (usually increasing it) often does the trick.

People have told me that thirty to sixty minutes after drinking the salt water they usually have an urgent and intense need to eliminate. This generally occurs several times over the next 45 to 90 minutes.

Some people gag on the taste. It's much easier to take if you use the non-iodized sea salt that Burroughs says to use. My wife recommends using a straw so that the taste isn't so strong or counting the number of swallows to take your mind off the taste. I have also found that the salt water flush is easier to tolerate as one's intestines become clean. People who have never cleansed often get a strong reaction. However, as they continue the cleanse, the salt water flush is more and more easily tolerated.

If all else fails, drink the laxative tea morning and night.

It's important to understand that there are two parts to this cleanse. Part one is the detox: mobilizing the waste from the parts of the body where it is stored. Part two is elimination: ensuring the waste is washed out of the body quickly and regularly so that the toxins are not reabsorbed, which will make you feel sick or miserable. The salt water flush is a powerful part of that elimination process.

Person No. 58

I did the herbal tea the night before. Then did the SWF the next morning. Why the diarrhea 40 minutes later? It's not explained in the book.

Person No. 18

Are you experiencing diarrhea or is the water just flushing through and taking the contents with it? The purpose of the salt water is to flush your digestive track and take anything present along with it. It normally takes about 45 minutes to an hour for this to happen.

Person No. 13

Yeah, I think a lot of people are mistaking diarrhea with what the cleanse is supposed to be doing.

You're breaking up the old feces and rotten plaque in your intestines. Then you're flushing it through with a lot of liquid. So, yes, the consistency is liquid, and yes, you are seeing brown. But, that is what's supposed to happen. This is cleaning you out.

You're replacing everything you need as far as nutrients and water with the lemonade, so there is no worry of being dehydrated as long as you are drinking enough lemonade.

Person No. 12

I wondered about this also, but it's normal as long as you are not having uncontrollable diarrhea all day long. I still have yet to have a solid mass.

Person No. 13

Yeah, nothing solid here either, which is fine with me. As long as I see something coming out every day, I know it's working.

Person No. 4

I have read the book at least twenty times, but I still have a question. Can I start off with the SWF (salt water flush) this morning if I didn't have a chance to do the herbal laxative last night? My last food consumption was six hours ago and it was just soup. If not, if I do the laxative tea now, how long must I wait to do the SWF?

Peter

You should not have any problem starting with the salt water flush in the morning so long as you have not eaten anything that day, even if you forgot to do the laxative tea the night before. Obviously it would be better to follow all the instructions exactly, but I do not think this is a serious omission.

The salt water flush should be done only when nothing else has been eaten or drunk before it that day. I know of only one person who has done the salt water flush in the middle of the day after lemonade and he was quite nauseated.

Person No. 34

I'm on Day 4 now. I tried the salt water this morning but could only chug down half a quart and then I felt like I was going to throw it all up. So I stopped. I had a tiny BM ten minutes after, but that's it. So, I think I'm just going to stick to the tea. I'm just not having any luck with the salt water. What about anyone else?

This second cleanse has been much easier for me. Last night my husband made homemade beef and vegetable stew. It smelled amazing. Normally, it would really upset me and my craving would make me so irritated. But this time I could just acknowledge the smell, recognize it was just a good smell and move on. I didn't have to associate it with eating.

Person No. 1

Due to this being my first ten-day fast, I am curious about how to get the internal salt bath to work properly. I am in Day 3 of my fast. I found the following site that mentioned exercises to make the salt water move quickly from your stomach to your intestines. Take a look. You may find it helpful. Please note that the site reference is for the salt water flush exercises only: www.lifeevents.org/salt-water-cleanse.htm.

Person No. 34

Wow, I just read your post on the salt thing and I went to the website and checked it out. Very interesting! I guess I'll give it another go. I hope I can get it right and it'll just work for me.

● Person No. 43

Okay, so I went out and bought the book at my local whole foods today and was so stoked on this whole detox that I went and drank the pint of salt water. Almost immediately, I had a sudden attack of heart burn and had an overwhelming urge to vomit. I'm only nineteen and I'm wondering what could have caused me to be hit with such a violent attack of heart burn. Could it be that I did the salt water flush about an hour after I had eaten?

● Peter

Yes, doing the salt water flush after eating is the wrong thing. The salt water flush should be done first thing in the morning after an herbal laxative tea the night before. [By the way, it's a quart of salt water (thirty-two ounces), not a pint (sixteen ounces).]

Person No. 43

In regards to the heartburn I had when I took the salt flush, I think the fact I used two tablespoons instead of two teaspoons caused my horrible discomfort. Today was my first day, too. I intend to try the flush again tomorrow morning.

Person No. 36

This is my first MC and when reading the directions I made note of all measurements. On the first day we did the salt flush first thing in the morning. Apparently I got up too early to try this and instead of using two teaspoons used two tablespoons of salt. Let me assure you that will flush you out quickly and very thoroughly. My wife is still laughing at me.

Person No. 59

I have a question about the salt water flush. Can you drink the salt water flush at night, say around 5:00 p.m., and then take the laxative in the morning? I drive a truck for a living so I work a lot of different hours and it is nearly impossible to do the flush in the morning. In the book it says to take the laxative tea at night and then do the flush in the morning or drink the tea again, but I would rather include the flush.

Peter

The only person I know who has done the SWF in the afternoon was nauseated by it. I don't recommend it. It washes everything in the system through and produces an urgent need to eliminate in about thirty to sixty minutes. At that point, it usually produces several bowel movements over the next hour. This would wash away the lemon and cayenne rather than letting it work overnight.

I recommend you just do the laxative tea morning and evening. It will probably make you eliminate several times during the day as well. I've never done it that way; I've always done the SWF. My daughter-in-law has done the tea morning and evening rather than the salt water flush and it's produced four or five eliminations a day.

Person No. 13
Well, I just started doing the salt water flush today. The reason I didn't start till today is because I wanted to see how it would affect me, and not on a morning when I had to work. Now I know pretty much what will happen and I can wake up early enough to deal with it properly. I plan to continue doing only the flush in the morning and the tea at night, because the tea seems to be hurting my stomach a lot. I might also try to find another kind. I am currently using Get Regular from Yogi Tea.

Person No. 8
I have a question concerning the amount of salt. I did the normal amount this morning and usually I have a couple of eliminations within the first two hours. This morning I went four hours before any elimination and then it was not very much at all. My question is should I increase the salt or decrease it? Thanks. Also, thanks for the bulletin board. It's fun to keep up on all of the replies.

Person No. 60
I'd like to answer Person No. 8. I think you need to use more salt. The flush should have at least the salinity of sea water. If it is less salty, it is not much different from soup—except for the taste—and soup does not produce eliminations.

It's the salinity of the drink that gives it the laxative effect. I read about traditional sea water enemas in some country that do the same thing, except of course the water is fed from the other end. I have used flushes from common table salt, not sea salt, and it works just as well.

If the SWF doesn't produce eliminations, it is not serious. However, you may find some of your body parts swelling a little. In all the cases I've known, the subsequent flushes produce the eliminations within a few days.

I can think of three reasons why a particular flush didn't work: 1) not enough salt; 2) too much food in the digestive track; or 3) the position of the food in the digestive track. If there is too much food to push to the end, one flush might not be enough. Subsequent flushes will take care of that. The flush works better if food is further down the digestive track. If the flush is done too soon after the last solid meal, it won't work properly. However, these are only problems with the initial flush. After you have been cleaned out, subsequent flushes should be alright as long as the amount of salt is correct.

Years ago, I came across a Japanese fasting method that uses Japanese soy sauce instead of salt. The recipe will make a drink as salty as, you guessed it, sea water. It showed me the flexibility of the system. Now, I use a dash of soy sauce with the salt water to make the drink more appealing. Especially when it's hot, it can taste like salty soup. A good soy sauce can give good flavor.

Peter

Soy sauce is not included in Burroughs' Master Cleanse and should *not* be added to the salt water flush. I want you to achieve all the benefits possible. The reason for not adding soy sauce is that it contains protein (amino acids), which requires significant digestive work. In addition, soy sauce is pasteurized and thus contains no enzymes to help with its digestion. It's like drinking steak or cooked meat as far as the digestive process is concerned.

Person No. 3

I am on day three and I have had no real BMs. Minor ones, but nothing I would consider detoxing. I am using the tea at night and I can only manage half of the salt flush in the morning. I read that increasing the salt might help, but if I can only handle half now, I don't think increasing it will help me. I drink so much liquid, I feel like I am floating. I am not hungry or craving anything. My only detox symptom is a sinus infection. I'm wondering if anyone had any suggestions, or ideas.

Peter

There's hope. Don't despair. First, be sure you're using non-iodized sea salt, not regular white salt. Sea salt is much easier to get down. I recommend Light Grey Celtic Sea Salt. Second, it is not uncommon for people who have been eating meat and dairy products not to have any solid eliminations for the first one or two days. Third, are you drinking laxative tea morning and evening along with the SWF? Until you are eliminating, drink the laxative tea both evening and morning.

Once you start eliminating, drink it in the evening only and do only the salt water in the morning.

Person No. 61
Is it normal to feel incredibly thirsty after the salt water flush?

Person No. 74
I am on Day 9 now and have learned that if I wait about thirty minutes after the SWF and drink another thirty-two ounces of water the thirsty feeling goes away. It also seems to help bring on the effects of the SWF super quick. Glad to know it's not just me feeling the thirst.

Sea Salt with Iodine

Person No. 4
I didn't read the label and bought sea salt with iodine added. Is this okay for the salt water flush?

Peter
I recommend that you follow Burroughs' instructions exactly because I know that will produce great results for you. Get non-iodized sea salt. I recommend Light Grey Celtic Sea Salt.

Shopping List

Person No. 47
Hi. I am starting the Master Cleanse this Thursday. I am very excited as this is my first MC! I am going grocery shopping tonight and was wondering if anyone can approximate how much of each ingredient to buy. Also, does anyone have a laxative tea they recommend? Thanks!

Peter
The only variable is the number of ten-ounce drinks you'll have per day. It should be between six and twelve. I've used eight in the estimate below.

The Master Cleanser book

At least 5 gallons (640 fl. oz.) spring or purified water (not fluoridated)

40 large organic lemons or 80 organic limes (or a combination)

At least 80 fl. oz. Organic Grade B Maple Syrup (usually sold in 32 fl. oz. bottles = 3 bottles)

1/2 pound non-iodized Sea Salt (I recommend Light Grey Celtic Sea Salt.)

2.5 ounces of cayenne pepper

A box of herbal laxative tea in bags (I recommend Smooth Move or Get Regular)

All of these things are readily available at most health food stores. Any herbal laxative tea will be fine. Some common ones are Smooth Move, Get Regular, and pure senna leaf tea. I recommend either Smooth Move or Get Regular as they are blends of 50% senna leaf with other herbs. Senna is the herb that is the usual main ingredient for herbal laxative teas. It stimulates the intestinal muscular contraction waves that move the food through the intestines. Some people find pure senna gives them cramps. That's why I recommend using one of the senna blends. However, you can also make half a cup of senna at regular strength and then add pure water so it's half strength. The only other option is mint tea.

By the way, most pure senna leaf tea boxes say not to have more than two cups per day and not to let children drink the tea. The blend boxes usually say not for children and no more than four cups per day. So watch that.

My wife and I guess it costs about $75 for one person for ten days. That is only $7.50 per day—not bad considering the amazing results available.

Sleeping Patterns

Person No. 6

Has anyone else's sleeping patterns been disrupted or is it just me? I'm on Day 6 of the cleanse, and although my body actually feels fabulous, I wake up at least two to five times per night to go to the bathroom. Is it the senna or should I stop drinking all liquids at a set time so that I can sleep through the night? Is this just normal? Help! Anybody got any answers out there?

Person No. 1

I did the toilet thing as well. If you did not eliminate that stuff your body would reabsorb the toxins and that would not be good. Do not quit. Just continue with the cleanse.

● Peter

You might want to be sure you drink the herbal laxative tea last thing at night as it takes six to twelve hours before it produces results in the early part of the cleanse and faster as you get cleaner. You may also want to switch over to a senna combination tea as senna is pretty strong by itself.

The idea of making sure you have drunk all your required lemonade by about 8:00 p.m. and then the tea about an hour or so later just before bed is also good.

I discovered that I'd fall asleep much earlier, say around 9:30 or 10:00 on the cleanse and get up around 5:00 to 7:00 a.m.

Person No. 12

I'm on Day 7 and I have no disrupted sleeping patterns, just strange dreams. I actually sleep better and wake up bright-eyed and bushy-tailed!

Smoking, Quitting During the Cleanse

Person No. 62

I am going to quit smoking January 1st. I am going on the patch. Can I do the cleanse while on the patch? Or should I quit cold turkey while doing the cleanse?

Peter

Burroughs says alcoholics, smokers, and drug addicts on the cleanse find their desire for stimulants and/or depressants goes away.

Person No. 9

Would it be a wise decision to just quit simultaneously with beginning the Master Cleanse? I know that sounds dumb, but it seems harsh to start a fast like that and quit smoking, although it does make sense.

Peter

Never having been a smoker, I cannot answer that except to say that quitting smoking and doing the cleanse has worked well for some.

Try it. If worst comes to worst, you could always go off the cleanse, quit smoking, and then start the cleanse again.

Please let us know what happens as it will be valuable information for others in your "shoes."

Person No. 6

I started the cleanse January 15th. And today is Day 2 for me. I was smoking up to two packs a day and drinking lots of beer. (I know I kept a couple of those companies in business.) At any rate, I decided that was it for me and this is coming from someone who tried to quit smoking at least nine times last year.

I have never experienced a more pleasant time quitting smoking. I think that my mind is so preoccupied with black forest cake, filet mignon and whoppers that I actually don't have much time to think about cigarettes and partying. In all of my fifteen years of smoking, I could never enjoy a cigarette on an empty stomach anyway. Good luck to you! I'm on Day 2 and guess what? I woke up at 5:30 this morning to go to the bathroom and realized something. I wasn't hungry! It just keeps getting easier and easier!

Person No. 61

Does that mean that smoking during the cleanse will severely compromise the results?

Peter

Like the rest of life, it is all relative. If you are a smoker and you are continuing to smoke on the cleanse, your benefits will be less than if you were not smoking. How much less? I do not know. Will it prevent getting any substantial benefits? I doubt it because we've had 110+ people do the cleanse in just this month of January and I believe that there must be smokers in the group who continued to smoke. Since I only know of about seven that did not get great benefits, I believe even smokers receive good benefits.

Person No. 63

My sister smoked while on the cleanse. Although she was unable to quit smoking, she did get tremendous benefits in other areas from the MC. Smoker or non-smoker, you will definitely benefit from the MC.

Spiritual Breakthrough

Person No. 12

Anyone besides myself have any spiritual encounters?? I had mine on Day 5. I felt Him deep, a feeling so unexplainable that I have never had before. I had uncontrollable streaming tears practically on my knees (weeping), along with some very, very strange coincidences and I don't believe in coincidences. I've always been a believer. I am now convinced about my beliefs and I am in complete bliss!

My first motive for this cleanse was weight loss; it has now changed to a spiritual motive. Let my new journey begin! I'd love to hear some more stories. God bless.

Supplements

Person No. 10

I have done the Master Cleanse several times and this time I thought I would add wheat grass tablets on the evening of Day 4, but cancelled them on the evening of Day 6 as my irritable bowel flared up. Too much fiber?

Peter

Thanks for the info on the wheatgrass tablets. That confirms what Burroughs says about not needing supplements on the cleanse.

By the way, Ann Wigmore, the person who propelled wheatgrass into the public mind, says that either chewing cut, live grass or drinking live, freshly made juice within a few minutes is the only way to use it. She says any form of cooking, drying or storing for a longer length of time reduces its enzymes and life energy to almost nothing. (I just read her book, *The Wheatgrass Book*.)

Tea, Other Kinds

Person No. 34

I know that occasionally we can drink mint tea to change things, but what about having a cup of green tea or any other type of tea?

Peter

Occasional mint tea and herbal laxative tea in the evening and optionally in the morning are the only teas Burroughs lists in his book. When you get to Day 8 or so, you will discover that whatever you went through was worth it.

Person No. 15

It's my second day with the cleanse and everything seems to be flowing smoothly, all puns intended. Thanks for this website. I've found it so very extremely helpful. I have a question concerning teas. I read in a bulletin that organic mint tea is an acceptable extra while doing the cleanse. What about, say, a lemon Rooibos? It's supposed to be very good for you, but I wasn't certain whether all teas are acceptable, or just the laxative and the mint. Any help would be appreciated. I'm going for ten days, wish me luck!

Peter

Hi Person No.15. I am not familiar with Rooibos tea. A search of herbal data on the Internet shows no references to Rooibos being a laxative by itself. There was one mention of Rooibos combined with senna as a laxative blend. That would be acceptable as it contained senna. Other than that, stick with the procedure as written, using an herbal laxative tea or mint tea for variety.

Tongue Coating

Peter

The coating on the tongue is something Burroughs mentions briefly. He says one of the best ways of knowing when the cleanse is completed is when your tongue is clean and pink. You will discover that it gets very coated during the cleanse.

I also had a furry tongue on the MC. I decided to continue the cleanse until my tongue was clear pink. It took twenty days. A friend did it and it took him twenty-six. The tongue does get coated with white cheezy stuff as you're detoxing. It does clear up if you continue.

Tongue color, shape and coating have been used for thousands of years in traditional Chinese medicine. It is quite amazing all the information that can be learned just from looking at the tongue! In case you are curious, here are two traditional Chinese medicine websites that talk about diagnosing the patient by tongue color and texture:

Person No. 2

I can vouch for the white tongue thing. I did ten days on my first cleanse and was only starting to get some pink back. I am on my second cleanse and Day 2 is a completely white tongue, headache for twenty-four-plus hours, and the salt water flush is a "pass through" with nothing in it. Last time I did the cleanse, on Day 3 there was an energy boost. I am hoping that will kick in tomorrow. The mint tea has really helped the way my mouth feels.

Person No. 21

This is Day 3 for me. I think things are going normally. I am definitely sleeping more soundly. I usually awaken in the middle of the night, but not the last night. I started the Master Cleanse with a cold and mild asthma, but now the symptoms all seem to be getting better without the use of medication. I think the cayenne is opening everything up.

Usually towards the end of the day I'm dragging badly, but last night I had a lot of pep. I did all kinds of chores and played with my two little boys after dinner.

I'm feeling tired this morning and my tongue is definitely "white." I probably just need to drink some more water. I ordered the MC book yesterday and I'm so anxious to have it. Good luck to all.

● Peter

Your white tongue indicates you are actually eliminating mucus in the intestines. The idea of the cleanse is to go until your tongue turns pink again, but not everyone has the time or intention to do it all in one cleanse.

Person No. 2

Day 9. Last two days have been great. I've put in nearly sixteen hour days, six hours of travel one day, lots of "mind" stuff. Tongue is not as pink as I would like, but it is better than MC1 (Master Cleanse the first time). I've lost eleven pounds as of this morning. I am ready to start back solely on raw food. I am going to only drink juices (got a juicer for Christmas) for about a week. I did not get my Day 7 aches, pains and massive detox like I did in MC1. I don't know if that is good or bad. I am judging just by how pink or not pink my tongue is.

Peter
I'm on Day 10 today and agree with what Person No. 2 said. This time (my fourth Master Cleanse) was much easier. It gets easier and easier. My tongue is nearly all pink! I'm also looking forward to raw food and juices.

I want to add wheatgrass juice to the raw food diet. From what I have read in Ann Wigmore's book, *The Wheatgrass Book*, juicing and wheatgrass are a very important part of four nutritional systems that appear to have helped patients with serious degenerative diseases for decades: The Gerson Institute (juicing, but not wheatgrass), The Optimum Health Institute, The Hippocrates Institute, and the Ann Wigmore Institute.

Peter
For the record, I ended my cleanse on Day 17 feeling great. My tongue went pink around Day 15 and then started to get a light yellowish-grey coating on the back part, but I ended it anyway. There's always another cleanse later. Friends and even strangers notice how healthy and happy I am.

My wife went through Day 15 and felt great also. Her tongue was pink with a light white coat.

I'm now eating raw vegetables, nuts, fruits, seeds, cold pressed olive oil, etc. drinking vegetable juices and experimenting with drinking one ounce of wheatgrass juice a day for a week. So far I've done three days of it. The stuff is vile. You are supposed to, and I have been, sipping it slowly and swirling it around in my mouth before swallowing. The first day it gave me light nausea. It's been a little better since. However, my tongue has gone stark healthy clean pink! I'm continuing my experiment.

Person No. 75
I read that the fast should end when your tongue turns pink again. Does this normally occur around the ten-day mark? I'm planning on doing it for ten days only, but if my tongue hasn't turned by then I guess I keep going?

Peter

For the record, the first time I did the cleanse, I went twenty days before my tongue was completely pink. It took a friend twenty-six days before his turned pink.

You do not have to continue until it is pink. You will still have some great benefits. However, for me and others I know, the wins from continuing until your tongue turns clear pink have included a realignment of priorities and goals, and more spiritual clarity.

Water Fast Only

Person No. 12

I am on Day 3 of the MC diet and I am doing fine. Is it ok to only have morning bowel movements? I am not going during the day.

I have stocked up on different fasting books to educate myself. One particular book *Fasting and Eating for Health* by Joel Fuhrman, MD states that any other fast or diet besides water fasting does not have the same effect or overall benefits as just water. I believe in the MC, but is there more research, studies or books to read about this diet besides Stanley Burroughs or your wonderful site?

Basically, Dr. Fuhrman, who firmly believes in fasting, is saying the organs can not sufficiently detox if you add anything to the water. I am slightly confused. I don't think I could do just water and I don't know how healthy or dangerous this would be.

Person No. 11

I would tend to think the opposite. On a water fast, you are definitely depriving your body of nutrients, whereas on the MC, you do "feed" your body by way of the lemon, syrup and cayenne. Also, don't forget that these ingredients are added because of their added benefits to the detox overall. For example, the cayenne will help loosen up the accumulated mucus, etc. I suppose people have their own preferences. I personally couldn't last on a water fast. I would worry too much about depriving my body of essential nutrients it needs to function properly. Anyway, I hope this helped!

Person No. 12

Thanks for the reply and yes it does help. I agree with you totally. I could never do the water fast. I am on Day 4 and still going strong.

The lemonade curbs my appetite and the water fills me up. I look forward to my tea at night, it's like my dessert. It's the salt water, ugh!

Peter

Person No. 11 is right in all he said and I'm glad you're doing well.

The one thing that health and medicine has taught me is that everyone is different. The same antibiotic that cures one will kill another with allergies to it. For the reason that everyone is different, I would say experiment and learn what is best for you. I am not interested in doing a water fast. I know two people who did and they had to have bed rest while they were doing it as they had no energy, but it might be good for your body.

The other thing I know is that more than 90% of the people I know who have done this cleanse the way it is written have gotten great benefits.

Weight Loss

Person No. 3

I am extremely interested in the MC. I have done some research on it and I am excited to try it. This week I have found that having a clear reason other than a diet is what keeps one's focus. With that in mind, I have read very little about weight loss and what effect/regaining occurs after the fast is complete, but what about it?

Peter

I was 6' 1" and weighed a little over 230 pounds in June of 2002. I felt terrible, too. My wife went on a 100% raw vegetable and fruit diet about six months before and after watching her getting healthier, younger looking and happier, I decided I wanted to feel that way too—even if it meant giving up foods that I really wanted (read "craved"). I spent six months eating only raw food and dropped to about 198 pounds eating as much raw fruit, vegetables, nuts and seeds as I wanted. Then on 4 Jan 2003, I started my first Master Cleanse. When I finished it on January 24, I weighed 175 pounds. I still eat more than 95% raw and have done the cleanse several more times since then and now weigh 165. (By the way, originally I couldn't fit in my size 40 pants. Now I fit comfortably in size 34 pants.)

So you can see returning to a solid food diet is not necessarily going to make all the weight return. Depending on what you eat after you finish your cleanse, you will keep off the weight, continue to lose more or put it back on. The cleanse does make one tend to want to eat healthier and does remove some cravings for those foods that are bad for your health.

I don't feel that people have to give up the "bad" foods completely, just realize they are not nutrition in any sense of the word, but fun. Just keep their consumption in perspective.

Person No. 16
OK, I stopped today after only eight days and I lost thirteen pounds. If I eat 100% raw food diet, with fewer nuts than veggies, and fewer veggies than fruit, will I continue to lose weight? It is important to me.

Peter
Yes, people lose down to their optimum weight (which is thin) while on a diet that is 100% raw veggies, fruit, nuts, seeds, sprouts, etc. Be sure to continue to drink plenty of water: one ounce of water for every two pounds of body weight and more if you are active. Also you need some sea salt each day as well.

Person No. 64
Hi. This is my first MC and I am on Day 8. I am following everything (the salt water in the a.m., Smooth Move tea at night and about ten glasses of the lemon drink per day). I have lost about four or five pounds so far. I am about twenty pounds overweight, so I do need to lose weight. Any ideas on why I am not losing much inches or weight? Are there other people that have run into this problem? I am eliminating and I have energy. I appreciate responses.

Person No. 13
The cleanse alone won't make you lose every pound you wish to lose. It's just a good stepping stone. You must continue after the cleanse by eating more healthy and exercising regularly. There are no shortcuts. This is just a good way to get in the correct mindset for doing these things. The fact that you are eliminating, losing weight, and have energy shows that you are doing the cleanse correctly. Look at the bigger picture. It's doing a lot more for you than just weight loss.

Person No. 64

Thank you for your response. You are correct. I have to concentrate on all the health benefits of the MC. It's just frustrating after not eating for eight days, not to have lost much weight, especially when others are losing ten to fifteen pounds. But, the big picture is important and that is why I went on this cleanse. Thanks for the support.

Person No. 13

You are welcome. You will reach your goals. Just take in a lot more raw fruits and vegetables, and get some exercise in. Start with any exercise and do it four or five times a week. As you start seeing results you will want to do more and do better. Being healthy is a lifetime process and commitment. It can be fun. It's just a matter of finding what works for you. This is a great motivational tool.

Person No. 65

Hang in there Person No.64. I didn't lose my weight until Days 11-14 on my last MC and then the third week of raw, the weight really came off. Do not give up now. You have come so far and it's doing your body such good to heal in this way. Stick with it and you'll be so proud of what you've accomplished, no matter what. Take care.

Person No. 64

Thanks, Person No.65. It's nice to hear that someone else took some time to lose some weight. I actually had only planned on a ten-day cleanse and today is Day 9. Based on what you said about losing at Day 11, I might extend a couple of days, maybe. As you said, the healing benefits are great. Thanks.

Peter

Keep in mind, Person No.64, that the excess weight is due to the excess fat that the body created to protect itself from the toxins. It will take a little longer to lose all the weight than it takes to lose most of the toxins. However, once you have lost the toxins, the excess weight will "melt" off rapidly.

Also, my wife found that although her excess weight didn't come off as fast as she wanted, she was still losing inches as her body changed shape because the fat deposits were disappearing.

Person No. 16

I'm between twenty and thirty pounds overweight and I am a strict vegan (and aspiring raw foodist). Today was supposed to be the first day of my second cleanse (I stopped two days early a week ago and so I was planning on doing it until the twelfth) but I came home and I couldn't resist the romaine lettuce. I would like to know what you guys think about how much weight I might lose in the next ten days if my diet consists of only laxative tea, our type of lemonade, and romaine lettuce with a light coating of organic soy and vegetable dressing. Thanks for any replies I get.

Person No. 1

I apologize for the long response below but I want to see you succeed with the Master Cleanse,

The Master Cleanse is a total body cleansing program. A few of its side effects are: the removal of internal waste, healthier internal organs, more energy, less toxins stored in the cells of the body, a cleaner, healthier digestive tract, the removal of mucus and hardened plaque from the body which is a precursor for diseases, a better body metabolism, a positive perspective regarding overall health and nutrition, and weight loss.

Speaking from my own experience with the MC, there are no quick fixes and magic pills for obtaining good health and a leaner body. What a person needs is patience, discipline, the right information regarding health and nutrition, wisdom to take this information and apply it properly and, most importantly, determination along with a personal reason that they want to be in better health.

You are on the right track to a healthier body and a better quality of life because you have chosen to do the MC Program. I would like to recommend that you do not modify the MC program so that you will get the positive results that you are seeking. By doing so, you will lose the weight and keep it off because your body will be free from toxins that cause your liver to not function properly, i.e. a sluggish metabolism.

I decided to do the MC because my metabolism was slow and my hormones were out of balance and I weighed 202 pounds. I was forty years old with adult acne. I walked four miles a day five days a week and I ate no processed foods or high glycemic foods and never lost a pound of weight. Something was wrong with that picture. I picked up a copy of *Natural Awakenings* and read Peter's article regarding the MC and this website.

I did the MC for twelve days. I should have gone longer due to the fact that it was my first time doing the MC. I realized that I have to be patient because one cleanse is not going to undo the effects of the past forty years of poor eating.

To make a long story short, I lost fourteen pounds. I properly broke the fast and am eating raw fruits, veggies and nuts. I have not gained the fourteen pounds back. In fact, I have lost three additional pounds. I took body measurements before starting the MC and my body's proportions have changed. Because I am eating raw fruits, veggies and nuts my body is still detoxing, just very slowly. My metabolism is functioning better than ever. I will do the MC three to four times a year as directed for the rest of my life.

Be patient. So what that you did eight days instead of ten your first time on the MC? Do not beat yourself up over it. Your body still reaped great benefits. Next time it will be a cake walk. Just mentally prepare yourself as to how many minimum days, hopefully ten, you are going to complete and just do it! Trust me. When you meet the goal of ten days you will want to go further. Just monitor your tongue color and listen to your body.

Good luck to you. If my seventy-one-year-old mother and I can do it, so can you.

Women's Issues

Peter
Since the first edition of this book, I have received several questions about continuing birth control pills while on the Master Cleanse. I have now heard from several women that they have not had any problems, nor has anyone mentioned any problem.

Person No. 76
How will this Master Cleanse interfere with a woman's monthly cycle? How many days should a person wait if at all?

Peter
Stanley Burroughs says that the lemon skin can prevent excess bleeding and clotting and that normal conditions will continue during menstrual periods.

Person No. 16

I had my period two weeks ago. I started again today, Day 1 of the cleanse. Is the cleanse to blame?

Person No. 66

It probably is the cleanse causing a flushing of the system. I have read that the body uses the period to cleanse itself. I found that when I do a major cleanse or change in diet that sometimes my period comes on sooner than expected.

If the flow is a normal one, there shouldn't be a cause to worry. If it is heavy, but you are not feeling tired, a lack of energy or weak due to the heavy flow, then also, don't worry.

Person No. 12

I have a very important question. I've been looking all around the web and can't find answers. I have been spotting this whole fast. I have never spotted in between periods ever. They are usually right on time. I had an ectopic pregnancy [pregnancy outside the uterus in the tubes] due to scar tissue in the tubes and a miscarriage from not producing some hormone.

Yesterday on Day 12, I experienced major, major cramps in my uterus. I don't know if it was me ovulating (sometimes I can feel it), but it was horrible. I also read it could have been gas in the uterus. I feel better today and had a semi-solid movement this morning. I am breaking the fast with fruit today.

Am I shedding my uterine walls? Can the scar tissue be releasing? Is this common? Do you think gas? I am still spotting this morning. I experienced these major pains while at work sitting upright. When I got home last night and laid down I felt ok. After my bowel movement I felt good too. Was it the colon pushing on my uterus? Help! Any websites, testimonials, books, etc., etc. will help.

Peter

I am not a doctor and do not have your medical data. So, I certainly cannot diagnose your problems. You will have to seek a professional or look within yourself. I believe firmly that every person knows the truth when they see or hear it. There is something in us that responds to truth, much like one guitar string starts to vibrate when another one is vibrating close by it. Along those lines, I will give you some of my thoughts, which I hope will help.

I believe that the spotting and cramps might have been due to the detox of your uterus, which may have been denied the proper nutrients and adequate supply of clean, pure blood for many years. Such a condition would have been brought about by years of very bad diet and no cleansing and could have been the reason for your ectopic pregnancy.

When someone detoxes, she often turns on conditions brought about by toxins as the toxins are eliminated on the cleanse. It is not uncommon for people with histories of rashes to turn on a rash for a day or two while on the cleanse before the rash goes away. This happened to a friend of mine on the cleanse two weeks ago. He had a history of hemorrhoids and on the second day of the cleanse, he had bleeding hemorrhoids. They were less painful than the times before the cleanse and eventually went away after a couple days. He thinks they are gone for good.

If your problems don't go away after a couple days off the cleanse, I would see a doctor. If they do go away, you might want to consider putting yourself on a health-restoring regimen for several months.

I believe such a regimen should include:

1) Not filling the body with more toxins as found in refined white flour and sugar products; meat; artificial flavors, colors, preservatives; alcohol; tobacco; dairy products, etc.

2) Detoxifying the colon to eliminate the toxins being reabsorbed by the blood and redistributed throughout the entire body. (The Master Cleanse is a way of doing this.)

3) Ensuring the body gets adequate good (non-tap) water (at least one ounce daily for every two pounds of body weight); non-iodized, unprocessed sea salt; and nutritional, raw vegetables (especially greens), fruits, sprouts, and soaked seeds and nuts to help the body rebuild the depleted nutritional reserves and organs.

4) Removing any stress-producing situations in the current environment.

5) Getting exercise and fresh air by lots of walking.

I did find one interesting article on the Web that I thought had relevance, "Why Are So Many African American Women Suffering with Fibroid Tumors" by Dr. Jawanza Kunjufu. Although it is about African-American women and I do not believe you are, the message is the same for any woman. Unfortunately, it is too long to include, but here is the address for you to read it for yourself: http://66.102.126.72/ Fibroid%20Tumors.htm. [Yes, I know it looks strange, but that is the web address.]

In his article, Dr. Kunjufu makes the point that poor diet can lead to fibroid tumors. In addition to direct problems, such as heavy bleeding and tremendous pain, over time they can result in backache, kidney obstruction and even miscarriages. He suggests fasting for one to three weeks; veggie and wheatgrass juice; exercise; daily enemas; herbs; and removing cooked food, meat and dairy products from the diet, along with meditation and prayer.

I think you have done a great thing for your body with the Master Cleanse. I believe it is more effective than coffee enemas and liver cleanses. Now you need to decide what to do afterwards. I hope this response helps.

Person No. 12

It helps a great deal, thank you. You are right, I am not African American but that article was helpful too.

The pain has gone. I will continue the salt water thing you suggest, good diet etc. I appreciate everything. I'm going to try to cross over to a vegetarian diet.

Peter

As regards moving over to a raw vegetarian diet, I have some suggestions.

Be kind to yourself. Do not beat yourself up if you eat some processed food. Just get back to what you know is healthy. If you find yourself in the SAD rut again, do another Master Cleanse. Each one will help you transition to healthy food more easily. The cravings for processed foods are just coming from toxins that can be eliminated.

Buy and read *12 Steps to Raw Foods* by Victoria Boutenko. It will tell you how to live with your friends and family whether they transition with you or not.

Find someone in your area who wants to do this with you. Having a "buddy" makes it doable. I know of several who have wanted to do this and tried, but they failed for lack of support. They had no friends to share stories and recipe experiments.

Finally, please post your experiences, recipes, etc. on The Raw Food Lifestyle board at www.TheMasterCleanse.com for others. We are the beginning of a huge movement toward true vibrant good health — without obscene cost. Thousands will come behind us and go through the same struggles. We can reach out a hand and help them by sharing our experiences, good and bad.

Person No. 12

Thanks again. Your support has greatly impacted my life. The valuable time that you share is greatly appreciated!

Afterword

Before time, there was and is understanding, peace, compassion, awe and bliss.

Good health is a reflection of that and as such cannot be separated from it, no more than you could separate the reflection of a flower from the mirror.

When we hurt, feel depressed or seem cut off from that understanding, peace, etc., it can only be because we have chosen to use our limitless power to conceal the ultimate truth from ourselves.

Joyously, the reverse is also true. Desiring, seeking, observing and acting are the keys which will always unlock our self-made prison door.

This book is dedicated to you and your good health.

For More Information

If you are interested in conference calls or one-on-one coaching on the Master Cleanse from the author or in possible future Master Cleanse retreats, please sign up for our free email newsletter at www.TheMasterCleanse.com. If you do not have access to the Internet, please mail your name, address, phone number and any particular area of interest to:

Peter Glickman, Inc.
PO Box 4984
Clearwater, FL 33758

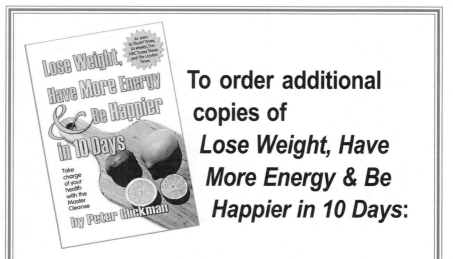

To order additional copies of *Lose Weight, Have More Energy & Be Happier in 10 Days*:

1. Go to www.TheMasterCleanse.com and click on the "Shopping Cart" link (all major credit cards accepted), or

2. Mail this form with a check or money order made out to Peter Glickman, Inc. to:

> **Peter Glickman, Inc.**
> **PO Box 4984**
> **Clearwater, FL 33758-4984**

Each copy is $16.95. (Florida residents add 7% sales tax.)

US shipping and handling is $3.50 (first class mail). Canadian & Mexican S&H is $7.00 (global priority). Other countries S&H is $11.00 (global priority).

Name: _____

Address: _____

City, State, Zip: _____

Phone: _____

Email: _____

(Your email address will not be shared.)

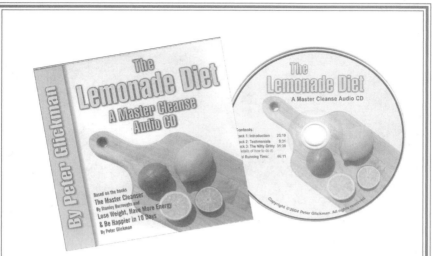

This CD by Peter Glickman covers the widespread nature of obesity, the body's method of handling toxins by creating fat cells to store them in, how to do the cleanse, and what pitfalls to avoid.

It's the perfect gift for people who would rather listen than read; especially good for your friends and relatives with questions about the Master Cleanse. Includes testimonial from a chiropractic physician.

Order your copy today. Go to the Web Store at www.TheMaster Cleanse.com, or mail a check with the form below to:

Peter Glickman, Inc.
PO Box 4984
Clearwater, FL 33758-4984

Each copy is $15.95. (Florida residents add 7% sales tax.)

US shipping and handling is $2.10 (first class mail).
Canadian & Mexican S&H is $7.00 (global priority).
Other countries S&H is $11.00 (global priority).

Name: _____

Address: _____

City, State, Zip: _____

Phone: _____

Email:_____

(Your email address will not be shared.)